Advance praise for *ManFood*

'This is just what the doctor ordered – Ian Marber has written the book every middle-aged man who wants to look after their health should read. It's the perfect antidote to the myths and misunderstandings that surround diet and health these days and gives men sound, evidence-based advice and tips. An excellent and much-needed book.'

Dr Max Pemberton, *journalist and author, www.maxpemberton.com*

'Finally, a book that tackles what men should be eating and how they can improve their health through food! For years the focus has been on everyone else. Now Ian has taken all that we know to be sensible and valuable about our nutrition and tailor-made it for men and their specific health problems. Men of all ages will find this book incredibly beneficial.'

Dr Ellie Cannon, *NHS doctor and resident GP for the* Mail on Sunday, *www.drellie.co.uk*

'There is an abundance of books on diet and nutrition available, each claiming to provide the ultimate panacea diet or promote the next health-food fad. *ManFood* differs in several important ways. It provides a logical and common-sense approach to the physiology of nutrition and the impact of our diets on our health. And, crucially, *ManFood* dispels the many myths behind supplements promoted as beneficial for men, by examining the scientific evidence for these claims. All aspects of men's health are covered, from the role of testosterone, through heart and gut health, to managing sensible and simple dietary changes and meal plans. *ManFood* is a book that finally gives men an authoritative text on evidence-based food claims, on how to eat healthily without gimmicks, and, most importantly, all expressed in the context of men's well-being.'

Dr Jeff Foster, *BSc MBCHb MRCGP DRCOG and GP with an interest in men's health, www.drjefffoster.co.uk*

About the author

Ian Marber is one of the UK's leading nutritional therapists and the joint founder of The Food Doctor brand. As well as working with numerous private clients, Ian conducts seminars, workshops and lectures, and works extensively with food manufacturers and retailers to develop healthy food ranges.

Ian has published eleven books on the subject of nutrition, and is a regular contributor to the national press, radio and television, including the *Spectator, The Times Body and Soul*, BBC radio, LBC radio, TalkRadio, *Mail on Sunday* and the *Telegraph*.

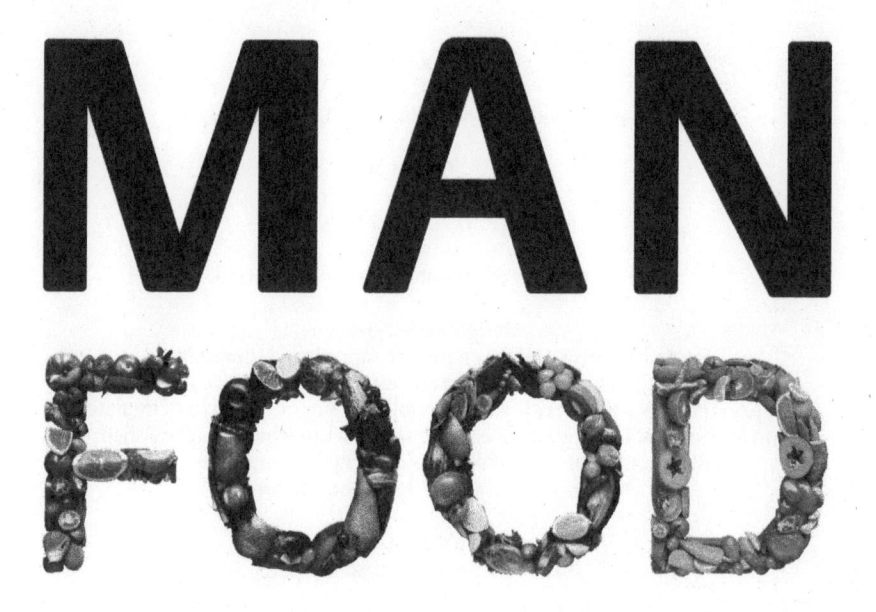

MAN FOOD

The no-nonsense guide to improving your health and energy in your 40s and beyond

IAN MARBER

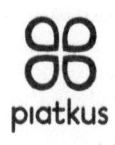

piatkus

PIATKUS

First published in Great Britain in 2019 by Piatkus

3 5 7 9 10 8 6 4

Copyright © Ian Marber 2019

The moral right of the author has been asserted.

A CIP catalogue record for this book
is available from the British Library.

ISBN 978-0-349-421643

Typeset in Albertina by M Rules
Printed and bound in Great Britain by
Clays Ltd, Elcograf S.p.A.

Papers used by Piatkus are from well-managed forests
and other responsible sources.

Piatkus
An imprint of
Little, Brown Book Group
Carmelite House
50 Victoria Embankment
London EC4Y 0DZ

An Hachette UK Company
www.hachette.co.uk

www.improvementzone.co.uk

Important Note
This book is not intended as a substitute for medical advice or
treatment. Any person with a condition requiring medical advice
should consult a qualified medical practitioner or suitable therapist.

For my godsons:
Daniel, Patrick, Oliver and Teddy

Contents

What is ManFood?

I qualified as a nutritional therapist in 1999 and have been lucky enough to enjoy a fascinating and varied career ever since. I have written several books and worked on television and radio, but the most enjoyable aspect of my job is conducting consultations. I have conducted some 6000 consultations. However, of those 6000 clients, only 400 or 500 were men. Given that I was one of the few male practitioners at the time, you might think that I should have seen more. Indeed, I often used to wonder, 'Where are all the men?'

It's much the same story on the radio phone-ins that I've been doing for the last fifteen years. About 90 per cent of the callers are women, while the few men who do phone the station tend to be young and ask questions about protein supplements and how to build muscle. Older men are much more likely to have health issues, so why aren't they calling?

In 2012, the University of Huddersfield conducted a study in which researchers created two diets. The first comprised burger and chips for lunch, followed by pizza and beer for dinner. The second was pasta salad and fruit at lunchtime, followed by rice with vegetables and a glass of wine in the evening. The 200 participants – who were more or less equally divided between the sexes – were asked to judge each diet for its perceived 'masculine' or 'feminine' properties. Regardless of sex, the second diet was judged 'significantly more feminine' than the first, and the men who opted for it were considered more feminine, too. The researchers concluded that such gender stereotypes may 'hinder attempts to improve men's diets if dietary recommendations are perceived as "markers of emasculation"'. I was amazed by this. Could it be true that men are not looking after themselves or making important dietary changes simply because they are worried about being perceived as effeminate? Could this prejudice also explain why they are not taking advantage of the health resources that are available to them? And is this a problem that afflicts just young men who feel strong pressure to assert their masculinity, or do older men suffer from it, too?

In attempting to answer these questions, first we need to consider men and their health. What comes to mind when you think of a healthy twenty-something? Are you picturing a shirtless, bronzed model with a well-defined six-pack on the cover of a men's health magazine? Perhaps you are imagining an elite sportsman, a famous personal trainer or a vigorous action movie star? It's increasingly common for health and fitness to be conflated, so it would be quite normal to think that muscle definition and fitness are the *only* manifestations of good health.

Now, though, let's try to do the same for a man from the next generation up – in his mid-forties or older. What comes to mind this time? It's not quite as easy to conjure up an appropriate healthy image, is it? A handful of action movie stars might still just about fit the bill, albeit with rather more wrinkles, but middle-aged male models tend to sport cardigans, as well as shirts, and most of the sportsmen have long since retired. By and large, older men are synonymous with pensions, Viagra and maybe the occasional round of golf, not health and fitness.

It's understandable that the media uses images of young people to represent good health – green juices and yoga pants for women, rippling biceps and abs for men – but this means that the older generations are often overlooked. And this is especially true for older men. While countless magazines and websites offer good health advice to women of all ages, men usually have to make do with articles about cars, sports and fitness (as opposed to health). Moreover, if a men's magazine does carry a health and well-being feature, it will generally be about the latest fashionable workout programme or popular diet, rather than something that will have long-term benefits.

In part, the magazines are merely reflecting their readers' interests, because men are notoriously reluctant to give serious consideration to their own health. For instance, in 2013, one survey found that British men who are not on medication are 32 per cent less likely than women to consult a medical professional if they suspect they have a problem. Two years later, another study reported that, while men feel the same emotions as women (of course we do!), we are loath to discuss them, especially with relative strangers, such as GPs. As a result, women are twice as likely as men to attend regular medical check-ups, and they are also far more inclined to take prescribed medication as directed. By contrast, a large proportion of men simply don't bother, even if they are suffering from a debilitating condition.

Similarly, women are more likely to avoid high-fat foods, eat more fibre and limit their intake of salt. They also eat less red meat and take fewer risks in terms of consuming undercooked food. To some extent, this may be explained by the fact that the diet industry focuses almost exclusively on women, so they have easy access to plenty of good information and sound advice on nutrition. Once again, though, men's apparent lack of interest in their own health is a major factor, too.

So, what's going on? Why are we failing to look after ourselves?

Take a moment to consider that prostate cancer has recently overtaken breast cancer to become the third-largest cancer killer in the UK (behind lung and bowel cancer). Deaths from breast cancer have thankfully been falling consistently since 1999, yet in the UK one man now dies every forty-five minutes from prostate cancer. There are several possible explanations for this, not least the fact that there has been far more research into the treatment of breast cancer than prostate cancer: literally twice as many scientific papers have been published on the former than the latter. We can only hope that more investment will start to address this imbalance, but men's behaviour and attitudes to their own well-being surely have a role to play, too. Prostate cancer can often be treated effectively, but only if it is detected at an early stage, so men's reluctance to attend regular check-ups is a significant problem. And the same is true of their indifference towards nutrition.

Research suggests that eating foods that are rich in carotenoids – which are found in brightly coloured fruits and vegetables – may reduce the incidence of prostate markers that are implicated in the formation of cancer. Similarly, sulforaphane, a chemical that occurs in cruciferous vegetables, along with green tea, a number of minerals, a healthy intake of fibre and omega 3 fats may also help to stack the odds against cancer. But how many men have even heard of these crucial compounds, let alone changed their diet to incorporate more of them?

Diet is also an important factor in the development of conditions such as heart disease and colon cancer, both of which are more prevalent in men than women. In addition, making smart dietary choices can help us increase our energy levels, offset stress, improve sleep, lose weight and regulate our hormone levels – all of which have major impacts on how we feel in ourselves. Yet, when we think about what men eat, our minds inevitably turn to boozy pub lunches, full English breakfasts, barbecues and takeaways. We really need to get away from these stereotypes as they aren't helping us.

Packaging and presentation might have a role to play here. A recent Canadian study reported that food packaging with clearly visible health cues (such as 'low fat', 'sugar free', 'rich in fibre') appeal to women, whereas men actively avoid them and gravitate towards foods that make no health claims. This may be linked to the cultivation of a certain type of masculinity among Britain's older males. For instance, I was born in 1963, and I was raised to view any sort of self-regard as a mild failing, and certainly something that 'real men' never considered.

Of course, this is a crazy, archaic attitude. We need to step up and take more control of our health and well-being. I have written this book to help us do just that.

ManFood is a food plan that ticks all of the boxes that relate to men who are no longer in the first flush of youth but still want to live healthy, active lives. It includes a variety of foods selected for their nutritional value and proven ability to reduce the risk of a number of serious health conditions. You'll find no gender stereotypes here, just plain-speaking, practical nutritional advice and guidance on how to eat well and enjoy all of the benefits that doing so provides.

And don't worry, while the *ManFood* plan is fantastic for your health, it's great for your taste buds, too. You won't find any recipes for kale smoothies in the pages that follow. Just dozens of great ideas that will help you live life to the full.

PART ONE

Health challenges for men

CHAPTER 1

Your heart

How to look after it

D o you remember how heart attacks used to be portrayed in the movies? It was always a man, clutching his chest, falling to the floor after a shock or major exertion. Later, if he survived, his family would gather around his bedside and tell him that he should have taken more care of himself. In a perverse way, they seemed to be *blaming* him for what had happened. I always thought that this was rather unfair, given how the poor bloke had suffered. But there is no denying that men are often their own worst enemies in terms of increasing their risk of heart disease.

I have one or two close family members who have suffered various heart-related incidents. In itself, this puts me in a higher risk category, so I pay particularly close attention to my cardiac health. But whether you have a relative who has suffered from heart disease or not, the statistics are particularly sobering for middle-aged and older men. For instance, the average age of first heart attack is 65 for men, compared to 72 for women. Similarly, researchers at the British Heart Foundation found that more than twice as many men as women in the 45–54 age group have circulatory diseases, and three times as many men as women suffer from heart disease between the ages of 55 and 74. One significant aspect of these statistics is that most people – men as well as women – are already well aware of them. Yet, while they may be familiar with the problems – such as the prevalence of heart attacks, strokes, high cholesterol and high blood pressure among Britain's ageing male population – they have very little idea how to address them.

Later, we will look at the crucial role that diet plays in either increasing or decreasing your risk of heart disease, but first we need to take a quick tour of the cardiovascular system to understand how it works and what happens to the various elements over time.

The cardiovascular system

The cardiovascular system is one of three components of the circulatory system. The other two are the lungs (known as the pulmonary system) and the veins and arteries (the systemic system). While these three components work independently of each other, they are closely related and are responsible for the flow of oxygen, blood, nutrients and hormones throughout the body. Any problems with them come under the umbrella term 'cardiovascular disease' (CVD).

The heart – a muscular organ that is a little larger than a clenched fist – first pumps deoxygenated blood to the lungs, where it is infused with oxygen before returning to the heart via the pulmonary vein. This oxygenated blood is then pumped to every other part of the body via an intricate network of blood vessels – the arteries and capillaries. The cells extract the oxygen for energy production before the deoxygenated blood travels back to the heart through the veins for the whole process to begin again. The average human heart beats about 100,000 times each day and pumps around 5 litres of blood every minute.

It's a complex and sophisticated system, but it can malfunction, resulting in some form of 'coronary heart disease' (CHD) – another umbrella term that encompasses a number of familiar health problems, such as heart failure, heart attack (technically known as myocardial infarction), stroke and atrial fibrillation (AF; the technical term for an irregular heartbeat). I shall explore all of these conditions over the next few pages, and explain why they are so strongly linked to diet and nutrition.

HEART DISEASE IN THE UK

- 7 million people in the UK have CVD, equally divided between the sexes.
- 42,000 people under the age of 75 die from CVD each year.
- 2.3 million people in the UK have CHD.
- 1 in 7 men die from CHD, compared to 1 in 12 women.
- 26 per cent of all deaths are caused by CHD (down from 50 per cent in 1961).
- CHD is now responsible for 66,000 deaths each year.

Source: British Heart Foundation factsheet, February 2018

Atherosclerosis

One of the most important causes of CHD is atherosclerosis. Each artery consists of three layers: an outer, fibrous layer that keeps the blood vessel in place; a middle layer made of flexible tissue; and an inner layer – known as the intima – that comes into direct contact with the blood. The space through which the blood flows – the tunnel in the middle of the tube – is called the lumen.

Over time, the intima can suffer spots of damage that attract a fatty substance called plaque. As these damaged areas grow, the arterial wall becomes less flexible (hence the term 'hardening of the arteries') and the diameter of the tube decreases (hence the term 'narrowing of the arteries'). When this happens, the pressure increases and blood flow accelerates. Imagine a garden hose that is furred up with dirt and gunk – the water spurts out of the nozzle at much greater speed and pressure.

Sometimes, the fast-flowing blood can start to loosen the lumps of plaque on the arterial wall. If a piece is completely dislodged, it joins the bloodstream and may eventually cause a serious blockage later in the system. The end result may be a myocardial infarction (if the blockage takes place in the heart) or a stroke (if it happens in the brain).

Men's risk of developing atherosclerosis starts to increase at around 45 years of age, whereas women don't reach the same risk level until the age of 55. (The difference may be due to the protective nature of female hormones, which decline during the menopause.) However, while there is nothing we can do about the ageing process, we can mitigate the risk by adopting healthier lifestyles and especially healthier diets. This is because obese people are far more likely to suffer heart attacks and strokes than those who maintain a healthy weight (see Chapter 5 for more details).

There's more to this than simply eating less, however. If you want to reduce your risk of developing atherosclerosis, you also need to eat smart.

Cholesterol

If you've ever had a blood test, then the GP probably measured your cholesterol level. They do this as a matter of course because there is a strong link between raised cholesterol levels and heart disease, especially after the age of 50. However, it should be pointed out that cholesterol is not all bad. In fact, it is vital to our health: it plays a vital role in the body's cell walls and is also used in the production of bile and a number of hormones. Indeed, we need so much of it that the liver actually manufactures it.

Cholesterol is a fatty, waxy substance, whereas blood is mostly water, and, as we know, oil and water don't mix. Therefore, in order for cholesterol to be transported in the bloodstream to where it is needed in the body, it is coated in a substance known as lipoprotein. There are several different types, but the two main ones are low-density lipoprotein (LDL) and high-density lipoprotein (HDL). The former is often described as 'bad cholesterol', while the latter is termed 'good cholesterol'. (It's easy to remember which is which: HDL for 'happy'; LDL for 'lousy'.) As you might expect, this is a massive oversimplification, but, as generalisations go, it's pretty accurate.

In short, HDL collects excess cholesterol that has accumulated in the body and carries it back to the liver, where it is broken down and then either reused or excreted. Meanwhile, LDL delivers cholesterol to wherever it is needed, so it's like a perpetual delivery and collection service. If the two lipoproteins continue to work in harmony, cholesterol does its job and the body remains happy and healthy. However, if levels of LDL start to exceed the amount that HDL can remove, it begins to accumulate in the intima of the arteries. What's more, the structure of LDL means that it is easily affected by other elements in the blood, which can result in further damage to the arterial wall through a process known as oxidation.

As mentioned above, cholesterol is also an important component of bile – a fluid that is used in the digestion of fat in the small intestine. After it has done its job, it is either reabsorbed into the bloodstream or excreted. Therefore, the level of cholesterol in the blood can increase if there is insufficient HDL to mop up excess LDL and/or if surplus bile is not excreted efficiently from the intestines. In addition, around 0.25 per cent of people suffer from a genetic disorder called hypercholesterolemia, in which the liver produces so much cholesterol that the body's reserves of HDL simply cannot cope. Medical intervention is required to treat this condition.

For everyone else, though, a few small changes in the diet can have a dramatic impact on the level of cholesterol in the blood. Contrary to what you might think, this isn't all about avoiding high-fat foods or even eggs. Indeed, it has much more to do with maintaining a healthy, efficient digestive system. This is because the level of LDL in the bloodstream is directly related to the gut's capacity to excrete surplus cholesterol. Thankfully, there are a number of simple steps you can take to enhance this, starting with increasing your consumption of fibre.

Fibre

There are several different types of dietary fibre, but for our purposes we simply need to differentiate between soluble and insoluble. The former combines with water to form a gel, while the latter remains intact, becoming bulkier as it absorbs the liquid. Many foods contain a mixture of the two, and both have their uses, but it is soluble fibre that is most helpful in reducing cholesterol. First, it ferments in the gut and combines with certain bacteria that prompt the liver to produce less cholesterol. Second, the gel that forms after it combines with water can inhibit fat absorption. Third, it binds to bile in the small intestine and so promotes its excretion, which causes the liver to manufacture more by extracting cholesterol from the blood.

On average, we consume just 18g of fibre per day, rather than the 30g our bodies need, especially as we get older. I recommend that a third of this should come from oats (see below), while the remaining 20g can be found in a mixture of pulses, beans, vegetables, fruits, nuts and wholegrains.

Oats

Like other wholegrains, oats are a rich source of both soluble and insoluble fibre: 100g of oats will give you around 11g of fibre. However, they differ from other grains because of the type of fibre they contain – beta-glucan – which is also found in shiitake and oyster mushrooms. This attracts cholesterol in the intestines, encouraging its excretion rather than reabsorption, and also provides some protection against the oxidation of LDL in the arteries.

Ideally, you should aim to eat around 3g of beta-glucan each day, which a small bowl of porridge or three oatcakes will provide.

Nuts

Most people believe that nuts are 'fattening' – a 1970s term if ever there was one. However, while they certainly do contain fat, it is largely unsaturated (see below), and they are a great source of fibre, vitamin E and phenolic acid – antioxidant nutrients that not only inhibit LDL oxidation but can also increase the body's reserves of HDL.

I recommend eating about 30g of unroasted, unsalted nuts each day (roasting harms their natural oils). That's about 20 almonds, 10 Brazil nuts or 15 cashews, ideally spread throughout the day. You may want to add some to a bowl of porridge for breakfast or have a few with an apple as a snack between meals.

Fats

The ManFood diet includes both saturated and unsaturated fats. These behave quite differently in the body, although they both have a physical structure that resembles a bicycle chain, with all of the molecules linked to their neighbours on either side. The differences between the two types of fat are due to the nature of these links. The molecules in unsaturated fats are joined together by two struts – known as a double bond – which means they are quite flexible. By contrast, the molecules in saturated fats are held together by just one bond, so they aren't so bendy. You can tell which is which because saturated fat (such as lard) is solid at room temperature, whereas unsaturated fat (such as olive oil) is liquid. The former is typically found in dairy and red meat, and it is widely used in processed foods, such as biscuits and pastries. Meanwhile, fish, avocado, seeds, nuts and their oils are all good sources of unsaturated fat.

These two types of fat have very different effects on cholesterol. Saturated fats tend to raise the level of LDL, whereas unsaturated fats raise HDL and protect LDL from oxidation. Therefore, saturated fat intake should be limited to just 30g per day. For reference, a matchbox-size lump of Cheddar cheese and a 200g rib-eye steak each contains about 20g of saturated fat.

Garlic

Garlic is a remarkably versatile member of the onion family that has a number of significant antibacterial and antifungal properties. It can also reduce both LDL and total cholesterol in the blood. If you crush it and allow it to sit for twenty minutes or so before use, this will activate its enzymes, enhancing its potency.

Hypertension

It quite common for blood pressure to creep up as we age. Indeed, many people – including some medical professionals – seem to accept it as a natural part of the ageing process. So, does it really matter if it starts to rise?

Well, high blood pressure, otherwise known as hypertension, can have a detrimental effect on several parts of the body, including the kidneys, the eyes, the brain (it is a risk factor for dementia), the heart and the arteries. For instance, increased blood pressure forces the muscles of the heart to work harder, which can result in them thickening, which in turn is a contributing factor to stroke and heart failure. For this reason alone, we should all aim to keep our blood pressure at a healthy level.

I'm sure you've had your blood pressure taken at some stage, so you probably already know that there are two readings – systolic and diastolic. Systolic represents the pressure of the blood as the heart beats, while diastolic is the pressure between heartbeats. So, when you have your blood pressure taken, the higher number is the systolic reading. This is measured as the cuff squeezes, a moment before it releases its pressure. Anything under 120 is considered healthy. Meanwhile, you should aim for something under 80 for the diastolic reading. These measurements are usually recorded as systolic over diastolic: for instance, 120 over 80 (written as 120/80mmhg). Doctors start to become concerned if systolic rises to 140 and/or diastolic increases to 90.

Hypertension is undesirable for both sexes, but it seems that men are more at risk from its effects in middle age for two main reasons. First, as mentioned earlier, the female sex hormones offer some protection that lasts until menopause. Second, men are less inclined to attend regular check-ups, so any potentially harmful increase in blood pressure may go unnoticed for a long time.

What contributes to hypertension?

There are several important contributing factors to hypertension, including:

- family history – you are at increased risk of developing hypertension if a close relative has it
- people of Caribbean and African origin are at higher risk than other ethnicities
- stress and lack of sleep
- being overweight
- salt intake
- alcohol
- high cholesterol
- smoking
- some medications
- other health conditions, such as kidney infections, lupus and sleep apnoea

As this list indicates, some of the risk factors – such as family history and ethnicity – are unavoidable, but that simply means you should pay even more attention to those you *can* affect. Of course, first and foremost for smokers is to give up as soon as possible. As for everyone else, the starting point should be to eat a more healthy diet.

Eat your way to healthy blood pressure

Salt
Maintaining a healthy balance between sodium and potassium is vital for managing blood pressure. In broad terms, sodium is found mainly in the fluids outside the body's cells, while potassium is found primarily inside cells. The kidneys extract excess

fluid from the blood and send it to the bladder for excretion, a process that relies on a finely tuned balance of sodium and potassium. If sodium levels start to increase, the kidneys find it more difficult to remove the fluid, which in turn means sodium starts to accumulate in the body's tissues, attracting water. The volume of blood then increases accordingly, so blood pressure rises.

As you probably know, sodium is one of the two chemical elements in salt (the other is chlorine), which is why anyone who is found to be suffering from hypertension is immediately told to reduce their salt intake. The human body does need *some* salt in order to function efficiently, but no more than about 200mg per day. Compare that with the recommended maximum daily amount (6g), and you will see that even those who observe the health guidelines probably consume far more than they will ever need.

We tend to think of salt as the stuff we sprinkle on meals just prior to eating them, but these days the vast majority of our intake has already been added to foodstuffs long before we even buy them. There are copious amounts of salt in all of the processed meats (bacon, sausages, ham), ketchup, mustard, pizza, burgers, cheese, roasted peanuts, crisps and even some confectionery (for instance, one very well-known chocolate bar contains more than 150mg). Therefore, if you want to cut down on your salt intake, you'll probably need to cut down on convenience and processed foods. To give you some idea of how much you might be eating even if you follow a relatively 'healthy' diet, a simple breakfast of toast or cereal, a takeaway ham and salad sandwich for lunch and fish cakes for dinner will probably give you upwards of 10g of salt – roughly double the recommended daily amount. This is why pre-prepared foodstuffs rarely feature in *ManFood*. If you make your meals from scratch, you'll be able to regulate how much salt you eat. If you leave it up to the food manufacturers, you'll almost certainly eat far too much.

Incidentally, it makes absolutely no difference if you favour fancy pink Himalayan salt, rock salt from the French coast, organic salt or regular table salt from a plastic bottle, sodium is sodium, and your blood pressure makes no allowances for provenance or price.

Potassium

As mentioned above, your kidneys can function effectively only if you maintain a delicate, healthy balance between sodium and potassium, so your blood pressure is likely to increase if you are deficient in the latter. It should also be pointed out that the health guidelines regarding the maximum daily intake of salt (6g) assume that you will get adequate potassium from your diet. However, increasingly, for many people, this is not the case.

Ideally, you should aim to eat at least 4700mg of potassium *every* day: it is excreted in the urine, so your reserves need to be topped up regularly. Fortunately, this is not difficult, as long as you eat a healthy diet, as it is found in virtually every vegetable and fruit. Butter beans, Swiss chard, sweet potato, spinach, avocado, tomato paste, peppers and bananas are especially rich sources, but in truth any fruit or vegetable will do, as long as you eat enough of them. Indeed, this is one of the main reasons why I recommend 'seven a day', rather than the familiar 'five a day'. For reference, 100g of broccoli provides 316mg, a banana 422mg, a medium-size sweet potato 542mg, two pieces of watermelon 641mg and 100g of cooked spinach 466mg. That's almost half of your recommended daily intake in five modest portions, so increase your consumption to seven, including some of the potassium-rich foods, and you'll be just about there.

In addition, many fruits and vegetables are excellent sources of fibre, which helps in the regulation of cholesterol (see above), and contain chemicals with potent antioxidant and anti-inflammatory properties, so there are plenty of other reasons to eat more of them.

Nitrates and nitrites

Fruit and vegetables are also good sources of nitrates. When these chemicals come into contact with saliva in the mouth, they are converted into nitrites, which in turn are converted into nitric oxide. This compound then encourages the body's blood vessels to dilate, which means the blood flows through larger tubes, so blood pressure drops.

Nitrates are found in lettuce, green beans, celery and rocket, although the best sources are root vegetables – most notably beetroot, carrots and radishes – which absorb the chemicals from the soil. Nevertheless, it is difficult to consume large amounts of nitrates by eating these foods in their natural states. Consequently, most of the research into their impact on blood pressure has given volunteers concentrated vegetable juices. Several studies have reported that drinking around 70ml (about half a wineglass) of beetroot juice per day reduced blood pressure by between 2 and 5 per cent, and juices made from other vegetables seem to be similarly effective.

When it comes to fruit, strawberries have the highest concentration of nitrates, followed by gooseberries and raspberries. On the other hand, high-fructose fruit juices can lead to an increase in fats made by the liver, so vegetable juice is probably the better option.

Finally, because of their dilatory effect on all of the body's blood vessels, nitrates not only enhance exercise and energy potential but also increase blood flow to the extremities, which can certainly improve quality of life, especially in middle age. I'm sure you can guess what I mean.

Homocysteine

You may not have heard of homocysteine, but there is some evidence that raised levels of this amino acid are linked to cardio-vascular disease, so it is worth discussing here. It is formed when methionine, another amino acid, is broken down. Methionine is found in many protein-rich foods, including nuts, beans, fish and eggs. As a result, it is quite normal to find homocysteine in the body, but it seems that high levels *may* be a contributing factor towards atherosclerosis, due in part to its potential to encourage inflammation. There is also some evidence that high levels *may* be linked to cognitive decline (see Chapter 3 for more details).

However, recently, a number of researchers have insisted that all of the evidence for a link between high levels of homocysteine and CVD can be attributed to bias and/or poor methodology in the early trials. They also argue that high levels are better explained by factors other than CVD, such as lack of exercise and excess weight. Indeed, at present, the NHS does not consider homocysteine a significant risk factor for CVD, so it does not measure it as a matter of course. Nevertheless, if you are interested in learning your level, you could arrange a private test. The optimal level is between 10 and 12 micromoles per litre of blood, but some people can register 100 or even more. Fortunately, if you take a test and feel your level is too high, there are a number of simple steps you can take to reduce it.

How to manage homocysteine

Reducing homocysteine is relatively straightforward and inexpensive because it entails simply increasing your consumption of just four nutrients – folate, B6, B12 and B2 – all of which encourage the conversion of homocysteine back into methionine.

Cos lettuce, avocado, asparagus, spinach, broccoli, liver and pulses, especially lentils, are all good sources of folate. B6 is found in high concentrations in poultry, red meat, offal, pulses, fish, whole grains, brown rice, cauliflower, peppers, chestnut mushrooms, root vegetables, melons and bananas. The best sources of B12 are animal products, such as red meat, liver, poultry, game, oily fish, eggs and dairy. Finally, B2 is found in dairy products, broccoli, spinach, red meat, oats, quinoa and rye. There are plenty of relatively inexpensive vitamin B complex supplements on the market, many of which claim to provide the full recommended daily amount of all of these nutrients, but I always favour increasing your intake through the food you eat, if at all possible.

It should also be noted that gut bacteria play an important role in the activity of many B vitamins, including all of those listed above, so eating foods that encourage the growth of beneficial bacteria is a smart way to raise levels. Such foods include sauerkraut, miso soup, kefir and yoghurt (see Chapter 10 for more details).

Statins

Statins are drugs that block the activity of an enzyme that plays a crucial role in the manufacture of cholesterol in the body. They also increase the number of receptors that sense the presence of circulating LDL, which encourages the liver to remove more of it from the blood. In addition, they can help to reduce the inflammation that is associated with the build-up of plaque in the arteries. Therefore, it's fairly obvious why doctors are so keen to prescribe them.

However, as useful as they may be, there is a lot of controversy relating to over-prescription and serious side-effects, including aching muscles, insomnia and digestive problems. Now, I'm no cardiologist, and every case is different, so I would never dream of suggesting you should simply ignore a consultant's recommendation to start taking statins. Nevertheless, I feel it is worth considering and discussing your dietary options first, rather than turning immediately to medication for a solution to high cholesterol.

CoQ10

You might not have heard of CoQ10 (sometimes known as ubiquinone), but if you look up statins and muscle problems on the internet, you will quickly learn all about it.

Like many other nutrients, CoQ10 – which is short for co-enzyme Q10 – has some notable antioxidant properties, but it also plays an important role in the maintenance of muscle tissue and cognitive function. The body produces it naturally, but unfortunately its capacity to do so starts to decline as we age. This can have a number of significant repercussions, especially in the heart, which may weaken and find it more difficult to generate energy as a result.

Moreover, statins appear to inhibit the production of CoQ10, which may explain why they are often associated with muscle fatigue and cramp. Consequently, you may feel it makes sense to increase your intake of CoQ10 if you have been prescribed statins. The highest concentrations are found in grass-fed beef, chicken, trout, sesame seeds, oranges, broccoli and oily fish, such as sardines and mackerel, but even these sources do not contain particularly large amounts. For instance, 100g of beef provides only about 3.9mg of CoQ10, and the same amount of chicken a mere 1.4mg. Compare that with several studies' recommended daily amount of 100–200mg, and you will understand that a much simpler option is to take a CoQ10 supplement. However, this will not be cheap: a daily 200mg supplement can set you back £30 a month. Now, you may consider that a small price to pay if it helps to alleviate debilitating muscle pain, but I advise discussing the potential benefits with your GP and a nutritional specialist before taking the plunge.

CHAPTER 2

The prostate gland

Why you need to get familiar with yours

D o you know where your prostate gland is, or what it does? A 2016 survey conducted by Prostate Cancer UK found that 17 per cent of British men know absolutely *nothing* about their prostate gland, while half don't know where it is and 92 per cent don't have a clue what it does. Given these alarming statistics, it seems a brief anatomy lesson is in order.

The prostate gland is about the same size and shape as a walnut. It sits just beneath the bladder and surrounds the urethra – the tube through which we urinate and ejaculate. Its sole function is to produce and store seminal fluid, the white substance that mixes with sperm to create semen. However, it may become enlarged, inflamed or cancerous – three conditions that can have a serious (or possibly fatal) impact on your health.

Prostate enlargement

Roughly one-third of men will have an enlarged prostate by the age of 50, while 90 per cent of 80-year-olds will have the condition. As these figures suggest, an enlarged prostate – technically known as benign prostate enlargement (BPE) or benign prostatic hyperplasia (BPH) – is an entirely normal part of the ageing process. It does not cause cancer and indeed is not even considered a significant risk factor for the development of cancer. Given that, what's the big deal?

Well, remember that the prostate sits around the urethra, so if it becomes enlarged, it can squeeze this vital tube. Therefore, an enlarged prostate is often linked to problems such as a weak flow of urine, difficulty starting or stopping urination, a feeling that peeing is no longer entirely in your control, and difficulty fully emptying the bladder. All of these symptoms can contribute to the need to visit the bathroom more often, especially at night, which can lead to sleep deprivation. Moreover, untreated BPE can develop into total blockage of the urethra so no fluid can get through. This extremely painful condition is called acute urinary retention and it will necessitate an immediate visit to accident and emergency.

Also, some of the symptoms of BPE mirror those associated with the early stages of prostate cancer, so it's important to arrange a prostate examination with your GP if you start to experience any of them.

BLOOD TESTS AND PROSTATE EXAMINATIONS

Every man should have his prostate checked on a regular basis, especially from middle age onwards. Most of us are familiar with the traditional digital rectal examination (DRE), in which the doctor inserts a finger to check for any enlargement, but this may be combined with blood tests to check kidney function and level of prostate-specific antigen (PSA).

PSA is a protein that is produced by normal cells in the prostate, but the level can rise with age, when the gland

→

is enlarged or inflamed, or, most importantly, when cancer is present. However, it also tends to increase after sex or exercise, when taking medication to combat hair loss, after a DRE, or if you are suffering from a bladder infection. Consequently, a significant proportion of PSA tests generate false positives, which have led to patients receiving unnecessary – and highly invasive – treatment, including surgery, for minor abnormalities that were unlikely to develop into serious conditions. In addition, the test fails to detect cancer in around 15 per cent of cases.

In light of these issues, many GPs are now cautious about recommending PSA tests, especially for men aged over 70, who are more likely to register a false positive result and therefore endure unnecessary treatment. Therefore, you should discuss the pros and cons of taking the test with your GP, then make an informed decision on that basis. I did this myself when I turned 50, but men of African or Caribbean origin, and those with close relatives with prostate issues, should consider having this conversation somewhat earlier, perhaps when they turn 40.

Alternatively, or additionally, you could enquire about multiparametric MRI scanning, which seems to be more accurate than the PSA approach and is becoming more widely available on the NHS.

The good news is that a healthy diet will provide several nutrients that can reduce the risk of developing an enlarged prostate and mitigate many of the symptoms that are associated with the condition. Three of the most important of these nutrients are vitamin C, lutein and beta-carotene (both carotenoids), which are found in high concentrations in:

- Egg yolk
- Kale
- Spinach
- Swiss chard
- Turnip
- Cress
- Green peas
- Brussels sprouts
- Sweetcorn
- Broccoli
- Carrots

- Sweet potato
- Peppers
- Peaches
- Apricots
- Cherries
- Oranges
- Melon
- Blackcurrants
- Kiwi
- Berries

Prostate inflammation

You may think that inflammation and enlargement are one and the same thing. However, while enlargement entails an increase in the number of cells in the prostate, and therefore an increase in its mass, the gland does not actually grow when it is inflamed – a condition known as prostatitis. About 15 per cent of men will experience prostatitis at some point in their lives, although it is most common among those aged between 30 and 50. But what causes the inflammation?

The most likely culprits are bacterial infections. These may be acute (i.e. one-offs) or chronic (recurring), but the symptoms are usually the same, including fever, fatigue, frequent and strained urination, a marked increase in night-time trips to the bathroom, lower back pain and sometimes sexual dysfunction. A visit to the doctor is essential if you experience any of these issues, especially as some studies have suggested a link between chronic prostatitis and prostate cancer. There is also an established link between prostatitis and sexually transmitted diseases – another good reason to get checked out. Both acute and chronic bacterial prostatitis are usually treatable with a course of antibiotics or antifungals.

Non-bacterial prostatitis, which is sometimes known as chronic pelvic pain syndrome (CPPS), requires the attention of a good urologist as it can be due to a variety of different causes, including such common conditions as stress, irritable bowel syndrome and poor gut health.

Prostatitis and nutrition

You may well have heard the welcome news that chocolate (or to be more precise the cocoa beans in it) is good for you, at least in moderation, as it contains bioflavonoids such as flavanols, isoflavones and saponins. Among many other benefits, these anti-inflammatory nutrients (sometimes known simply as flavonoids) seem to be highly effective at reducing the risk of prostatitis.

In total, there are some 6000 different flavonoids, and they are found in just about every foodstuff that isn't animal in origin. For instance, every time you eat an apple or a banana, you'll benefit from their flavanols. High concentrations of flavonoids are also found in quinoa, rye bread, chickpeas, Brazil nuts, sesame seeds, walnuts, rice and wheat. Therefore, simply eating your five (or, preferably seven) a day will almost certainly help you combat inflammation of the prostate.

On the other hand, you should avoid caffeine, alcohol, spicy food and especially chilli peppers if you have been diagnosed with prostatitis as these are all liable to irritate an already bothered bladder.

Prostate cancer

Of course, prostate cancer has the potential to affect only half of the population, yet it is now the third most common cancer in the UK, just behind lung and bowel cancer. The 47,000 new cases diagnosed in 2015 represented 13 per cent of all cancers, and there has been a 44 per cent increase in diagnosed cases since the 1990s. Although 84 per cent of those who are diagnosed with the disease survive for ten years or more, there were still in excess of 11,500 prostate cancer deaths in 2016. That's more than six times the number of people who die on the UK's roads each year. To put it another way, approximately 31 British men die of prostate cancer every day.

Some men are at greater risk of developing the disease than others, yet one survey found that 88 per cent of those men are unaware of the fact. For instance, your risk increases significantly if a parent or sibling has suffered either prostate or breast cancer, and the disease affects one in four black men, compared to only one in eight white. If you are in one of these high-risk groups, it is imperative to maintain an ongoing dialogue with your doctor and report any changes in your general well-being and especially any bladder problems. This is even more important later in life, as risk is closely related to age. At present, many men are dying needlessly, because 40 per cent of cases are diagnosed at a late stage, when treatment is much less likely to prove effective.

The most likely cause of urinating more often, weak flow or a sudden urge to pee is BPE, but it's always best to check with your doctor, especially if you suffer pain during urination. Remember that the urethra runs straight through the prostate gland, so any sort of growth – including a cancerous tumour – can press on the tube and have an impact on urination. Traces of blood in the semen, pelvic and/or back pain and inexplicable weight loss should also be investigated as soon as possible.

As mentioned above, the level of PSA in the blood usually increases if cancer is present, but this test is far from infallible. A very slow-growing mass may go undetected for life, or a test may indicate normal PSA just before a highly aggressive tumour starts to expand.

Risk factors

It goes without saying that the pathology of all cancers – including their formation and progression – is highly complex. While several long-term studies have identified a number of risk factors over which we all have some control, no one can guarantee that they will remain cancer free throughout their life. Nevertheless, there are some simple steps that are likely to reduce your risk of developing the disease, and help you feel healthier in the process.

Weight
Overweight and obese people are at greater risk of developing many of the most common cancers, including prostate. In addition, excess weight seems to increase both the risk of recurrence and the likelihood of contracting particularly aggressive forms of the disease. See Chapter 5 for detailed advice on how to lose weight while maintaining good nutrition.

Dairy products and calcium
Many people routinely take a multivitamin supplement that includes 100 per cent of the recommended daily amount of calcium, presumably because of this mineral's fabled ability to protect against osteoporosis later in life. However, unless they are vegan, they are likely to get more than enough simply from eating and drinking dairy products. Moreover, there is mounting evidence that excessive consumption of calcium and/or dairy products may not be so healthy after all.

Much of the research in this field revolves around a hormone called insulin growth factor (or IGF-1). This is made naturally in the human body, where it plays a vital role in building and maintaining bone and tissue, especially in the early years of life. It is also found in high concentrations in cow's milk, where it serves the useful purpose of promoting rapid growth in calves. However, a number of studies have suggested that elevated levels of IGF-1 in the human body – possibly due to excessive consumption of dairy products – may also stimulate the growth of cancerous cells.

Meanwhile, other scientists have claimed that it is not the presence of the hormone itself but the protein-rich nature of dairy products that causes the problem, given that protein stimulates the production of IGF-1 in the body. Either way, excessive consumption of dairy does seem to be linked to elevated IGF-1 in the blood, which in turn seems to increase the likelihood of developing prostate cancer.

On the other hand, a third group of scientists have gone down a different route and argue that we don't need to worry about the IGF-1 or the protein in dairy products. Instead, we should be more concerned about the calcium.

In addition to maintaining bone density, this mineral plays a vital role in blood clotting, the transmission of signals between nerves, muscle contraction and many other important bodily functions. Therefore, men under 55 are advised to consume 700–800mg per day, while those over 55 should aim for 1200mg, which may seem a lot when compared with other RDAs. However, just four modest servings of dairy products each day are more than enough to provide this amount, especially as calcium is also found in kale, chicken, lettuce, beans and pulses, almonds, sesame seeds and many other foodstuffs. (Milk with porridge or in a mug of tea or coffee, a matchbox-sized lump of cheese or a small pot of yoghurt is one serving.)

Although the research is far from conclusive, I would advise sticking to this limit as there is sufficient evidence to suggest that excessive consumption of calcium – especially in dairy form – might be linked to a slightly increased risk of developing prostate cancer. And you should certainly not need to take a calcium supplement if you follow the ManFood plan.

Cholesterol

Most people are aware of the link between cholesterol and heart health (see Chapter 1 for more details), but many studies have also connected it to prostate cancer. As yet, it has proved impossible to establish which comes first – the cholesterol or the cancer – but you have nothing to lose, and possibly plenty to gain, by getting your cholesterol under control, especially as the link to the most aggressive forms of the disease seems to be particularly strong. Following the ManFood plan will help you achieve this.

Prostate-healthy foods

I have already mentioned several of the nutrients that can reduce the risk of developing an enlarged prostate, inflammation and cancer, or mitigate the symptoms if you already have one of these conditions. Now it's time to discuss them in more detail.

Carotenoids and vitamin C

Carotenoids are fat-soluble nutrients that give some foods their red, yellow or orange colour. There are over 600 different types, but those that occur most commonly in diets that are rich in fruit and vegetables are alpha-, beta- and gamma-carotene, beta-cryptoxanthin, lutein, lycopene and zeaxanthin. All of these carotenoids have impressive antioxidant properties, which means that they counteract the harmful process of oxidation that can damage cells.

Most of the attention with respect to prostate cancer has focused on lycopene, which seems to offer a worthwhile degree of protection against the disease. It is found in many fruits and vegetables, including red pepper, guava and watermelon, but tomatoes have the highest concentration. Moreover, the digestive system finds it easier to absorb lycopene when it is warmed, which makes cooked tomatoes the ideal source. In addition, tomato sauce, passata, paste and purée all provide just as much, if not more, lycopene as the raw fruit. Unsurprisingly, then, these are staples of the ManFood plan.

Pomegranate also contains lycopene, along with flavonoids, and some studies have claimed that its juice helps to keep PSA at a healthy, low level. Unfortunately, all of the research is based on drinking around a litre a day, which is probably unsustainable, but a small glass once a day may provide a certain amount of protection, and certainly will do no harm.

Beta-carotene seems to offer a degree of protection, too. It is found in sweet potato, pumpkin, spinach, squash, apricots and many other brightly coloured foodstuffs, and in this instance absorption is not aided by cooking.

Vitamin C is also found in nearly all foods that contain carotenoids, and there is mounting evidence that this is associated with reduced risk of prostate cancer.

Indole-3 carbinol and sulforphane

Although they sound like they belong in a lab, indole-3 carbinol and sulforphane are natural plant chemicals that are found mostly in cruciferous vegetables, such as broccoli, Brussels sprouts, kale, pak choi and cauliflower. Research suggests that increased intake of these products not only inhibits the spread of prostate cancer in its early stages but also reduces the risk of developing aggressive forms of the disease in the first place. Interestingly, these foods also usually contain selenium, which makes them even better allies in the battle against prostate cancer.

Selenium

Selenium is a mineral that is found in small quantities in fish such as tuna, herring, halibut, cod, salmon and mackerel as well as Brazil nuts, walnuts, cashews, oats, brown rice, barley, offal, chicken and button mushrooms. Research has shown that all of these foods may help to reduce the risk of prostate cancer because selenium is an important component of a powerful antioxidant called glutathione peroxidase. However, they should be eaten in moderation. The recommended daily amount, or RDA, is a tiny 55mcg daily, while the maximum safe intake is just 400mcg per day. Therefore, you should be careful if you are particularly fond of any of these foods, as high intake over a prolonged period of time could actually promote, rather than reduce, oxidation. For the same reason, you should always seek medical advice before taking a selenium supplement.

It should be noted that a single Brazil nut may contain as much as 75mcg of selenium, so just two will provide almost three times the RDA.

Catechins

Two types of catechin – epicatechin (EC) and epigallocatechin gallate (EGCG) – are found in high concentrations in green, white and oolong teas, all of which are commonly drunk in Asia. Meanwhile, they are found in much smaller quantities in the black tea that is favoured in the West. As a result, there have been extensive studies of these flavonoids, primarily because the rates of prostate cancer tend to be far lower in Asia, and researchers have speculated that this may be due to the locals' preference for green tea. Thus far, the results have been encouraging, as it seems that both EC and EGCG may inhibit histone deacetylases – a protein that is found in cancerous cells.

Therefore, regular daily intake of unsweetened and unsalted green tea may offer some protection against cancer, especially for those who are deemed to be at high risk of developing the disease. Most of the studies suggest a minimum of six cups per day to achieve a significant effect, which may sound a lot, but it is entirely feasible if you substitute green tea for most (if not all) of your usual cups of black tea and coffee.

Vitamin D

Most people are aware of the importance of vitamin D, which is manufactured when the skin is exposed to sunlight and plays an essential role in helping the body to absorb calcium. Some researchers have also claimed that it may counteract prostatitis and even slow the progression of prostate cancer, although it should be said that the largest study into vitamin D and cancer found no evidence of any link between the two.

Nevertheless, there is no downside to increasing your supply of vitamin D, especially in the depths of the British winter, when the body struggles to make as much as it needs. Portobello mushrooms are one of the few good food sources, especially when they are exposed to sunlight before eating, and it is also found in oily fish, egg yolks and dairy products. However, it can be difficult to get sufficient quantities from diet and sunlight alone, so this is one of the few instances when I recommend routine supplementation (see Chapter 16 for further details).

Isoflavones

Soya contains a number of isoflavones that bind to the body's oestrogen receptors and seem to offer some protection against contracting several forms of cancer, including prostate. Soya milk is well established as one of the main alternatives to cow's milk, while tofu, soya yoghurt and edamame beans (which are simply immature soya beans in the pod) are also widely available. Adding these foodstuffs to your diet will mean you will reap the benefits of nutrients that are hard to find elsewhere.

Ursolic acid

We've all heard the expression 'An apple a day keeps the doctor away', but what about the benefits of apple *peel*? Ursolic acid is a waxy plant chemical that is found in apple skins, rosemary and thyme, and a number of studies have suggested that this chemical may counteract BPE and slow the progression of cancerous cells in the prostate. Although much of this research has involved injecting ursolic acid directly into the bloodstream, there is every reason to believe that simply adding a few apples to your diet may be similarly beneficial.

Supplements

If possible, you should always to try get the nutrients your body needs from the food you eat, rather than bottles of pills. This is because the vitamins, minerals and other nutrients in foodstuffs are often more than the sum of their parts, as they interact with one another to provide additional benefits. Consequently, I recommend supplementation only in very specific circumstances (for instance, to boost levels of vitamin D during the winter).

As for alleviating the symptoms of BPE, three supplements merit consideration:

1. Saw palmetto is a plant that is found in the south-east of the United States, and its concentrated fruit extract is widely recommended by alternative health practitioners for the treatment of BPE. However, one meta-analysis of a number of scientific papers found that this had no significant impact on the lower urinary tract symptoms that usually accompany an enlarged prostate or prostatitis. On the other hand, a couple of other papers have found some evidence of its efficacy in the mitigation of both conditions.
2. Quercetin, a flavanol that is found in apples, peppers, capers, onions, dark berries and cruciferous vegetables, is a powerful anti-inflammatory, so it could be useful in combating prostatitis.
3. As we have seen, lycopene, catechins and sulforphane are three of the more important nutrients in maintaining good prostate health, and all three are available in a single capsule.

It is feasible that all three of these supplements *might* be beneficial . . . if you are prepared to take them religiously for the rest of your life. But is that likely? Many people buy a bottle with the best of intentions, take the pills every day, feel no discernible benefit, then never bother again.

Then there's the cost. The average price of saw palmetto capsules is about £10 for a 90-day supply (£40 a year), quercetin is generally about £10 a month (£120 a year), while the combination lycopene/catechins/sulforphane capsules are an eye-watering £19 a month (£228 a year). That's almost £400 a year. Now, you may think that is a small price to pay to *guarantee* a healthy prostate for the rest of your life, but none of these supplements actually makes that claim. (Indeed, all of the available evidence suggests they would leave themselves open to ruinous litigation if they did.) And where does it stop? We haven't even mentioned green tea extract and probiotics yet.

As you have to eat anyway, it makes much more sense to increase your supply of all of these beneficial nutrients through your *food* – that's what the ManFood plan is all about.

CHAPTER 3

Cognitive function and dementia

Don't bury your head in the sand

Lifestyle improvements and medical advances mean that life expectancy is increasing. I was born at the end of 1963, and at that time the life expectancy of a newborn male was just 71.13 years. Compare that with a boy born in 2016, who can expect to live for 79.2 years, with a 21 per cent chance of making it to 90.

However, while a long life is all very well, it becomes much less attractive if it is accompanied by serious physical and mental decline. Today, one of the greatest challenges we face is an ageing population with increasing incidence of Alzheimer's disease and other forms of dementia. Many people worry about the prospect of mental decline, but at the same time they are far from sure what they can do about it, if anything.

Dementia is a loose umbrella term that is used to describe a general decline in brain function. Any one of several conditions may cause it, but many of them are associated with a build-up of proteins within the brain, which in turn leads to a reduction in the number of brain cells. The Alzheimer's Society describes these conditions as 'usually progressive and eventually severe'.

Alzheimer's itself is by far the most common form of dementia, accounting for 62 per cent of diagnosed cases. By contrast, vascular dementia accounts for just 17 per cent of cases. The remainder are classified as suffering from 'mixed dementia' – a combination of two or more types. All of these conditions are characterised by memory loss, confusion and problems with speech and comprehension.

In the UK, an estimated 850,000 people were suffering from dementia in 2018, but this figure was expected to rise to over a million by 2025. One in six people over the age of 80 are currently affected, although some 40,000 under the age of 65 are living with dementia, too. Sixty-five per cent of sufferers are women, but this may simply reflect the fact that women tend to live longer than men. Of course, the disease also has a profound impact on partners and families, as they have to deal with the anguish of providing care for someone who may not even recognise them by the time the dementia reaches its advanced stages.

As these statistics imply, anyone can develop dementia, and the risk increases exponentially as we age. However, there is growing evidence that some fairly simple adjustments to diet and lifestyle can help to reduce that risk.

Alzheimer's

Alzheimer's disease currently accounts for some 8 per cent of all male deaths in the UK, meaning it is now the second most common cause of death, behind heart disease. It is caused by the build-up of two substances in the brain – plaque and tangles. Plaque consists of a sticky protein called beta-amyloid that blocks the signals between neurons in the brain and may also lead to harmful inflammation. Inside these damaged nerve cells, the fibres of another protein called tau become twisted to form tangles, which hinder the movement of nutrients into the cells. Both of these proteins are present in very high concentrations in people suffering from Alzheimer's disease.

One of the first areas of the brain to be affected by plaque and tangles is the hippocampus. Initially, this affects memory formation, so a sufferer may struggle to store new memories. Hence, they are likely to forget what they have just said or done. By contrast, older memories often remain unaffected at first, as these have already been stored in other, undamaged parts of the brain. The amygdala is often damaged in the next stage of the disease. This part of the brain has a significant role to play in feelings and emotions, so sufferers may start to make seemingly inappropriate, tactless or rude comments.

Vascular dementia

As neurons require a constant supply of oxygen and nutrients, any interruption, such as one caused by a stroke, has the potential to change the way we function. If the particular part of the brain that is affected is responsible for language, memory or cognition, the subsequent condition is termed vascular dementia. It should be noted that this condition is not necessarily caused by one single, catastrophic event, such as a major stroke. Indeed, it is more likely to be due to the cumulative effect of dozens of mini-strokes – technically known as transient ischemic attacks (TIAs) – each of which may be barely noticeable to the individual concerned.

The most common cause of vascular dementia is so-called 'small vessel disease', which entails a gradual narrowing of the blood vessels deep inside the brain. Therefore, both prevention and treatment are very similar to the approaches that are recommended for cardiovascular disease (see Chapter 1 for more details).

Risk factors for dementia

Hypertension

The link between hypertension (high blood pressure) and vascular dementia – and indeed Alzheimer's – is well established. Several studies have shown that raised blood pressure between the ages of 40 and 64 increases the risk of developing dementia later in life. This is hardly surprising as hypertension increases the risk of stroke, contributes to thickening of the blood vessel walls and reduces the diameter of the lumen (resulting in a vicious circle of ever-increasing blood pressure). This process can occur anywhere in the body, but the hippocampus seems to be particularly susceptible to it.

There are several possible reasons why hypertension may be linked to cognitive decline, including an increase in plaque and tangles, reduced blood flow to the hippocampus, and damage to micro-vessels deep within the brain. Maintaining healthy blood pressure, especially from middle age onwards, reduces the likelihood of all of these problems developing.

Cholesterol

A number of studies have found that high cholesterol in middle age is associated with greater incidence of vascular dementia and Alzheimer's later in life. The precise nature of this link is unclear, although there seems to be an especially close association between cholesterol and beta-amyloid, the main constituent of plaque.

There is one type of cholesterol, 24S-hydroxycholesterol, the result of degraded neurones, that has been found to be higher in sufferers of vascular dementia and Alzheimer's. With that in mind, it makes sense to maintain a low, healthy level of cholesterol in order to reduce your risk of developing Alzheimer's and dementia, as well as a number of cardiovascular conditions. However, there is considerable debate about whether statins are the best course of action to achieve this, given that several studies have found little or no evidence that these drugs reduce either the incidence or the progression of dementia. I recommend asking your GP for further advice.

Dietary fats

Back in the 1970s, the theory was that all fats should be limited or even avoided. This dictum persisted for more than thirty years, so it probably played a significant role in the way you think about food and nutrition. Maybe you grew up hearing adults saying that you should never eat chicken skin and should always trim the fat off steak? Recently, researchers have started to challenge these ideas, but what about the most vilified fat of all – saturated fat? Surely we should continue to avoid *that*, shouldn't we?

The short answer is 'Yes, but limit rather than cut out.' The evidence is far from conclusive either way, but a majority of studies suggest that saturated fat may play some sort of role in the development of dementia and cognitive decline. And similar accusations have been levelled against trans fats. These are normal vegetable fats that are chemically altered by the addition of hydrogen ions. This process makes them much less flexible than the original, natural fats, so they are solid at room temperature. This made them very useful for the food industry, which once used them extensively in baked goods, such as biscuits and cakes, fried foods, frozen pizzas and other highly processed foods. They are less common nowadays, but they have not been eradicated entirely. You are probably familiar with the terms 'hydrogenated vegetable oil', 'hydrogenated fat' and 'partially hydrogenated fat', all of which are trans fats.

Some studies have suggested that trans fats can find their way into the structure of cells and then reduce their ability to communicate with one another, which is obviously a very serious issue if it happens in neurons. They have also been linked with raised levels of cholesterol, another risk factor for dementia (see above).

Omega 3

Omega 3 is one of a number of beneficial fats (sometimes called essential fats) that are found in a variety of foodstuffs. There are three different forms of omega 3: alpha linolenic acid (ALA), which is found in flaxseed, chia seeds and walnuts, among other nuts and seeds, and eicosapentaenoic acid (EPA) and docosahexaenoic acid (DHA), both of which are found in high concentrations in oily fish, such as mackerel, salmon and herring, as well as other marine foods.

All of these compounds have been subjected to extensive research in relation to their ability to mitigate cognitive decline. Approximately 85 per cent of the studies into omega 3 obtained from food sources have reported beneficial effects on the brain, compared with only 61 per cent of trials that have studied the impact of supplements. In addition, one study reported significant benefits when older people who had already been diagnosed with dementia increased their intake of omega 3 foodstuffs. Once again, this suggests that you should always try to get the nutrients you need from food, rather than a capsule.

All three types of omega 3 have anti-inflammatory properties, play an important role in cell structure and help to combat both high cholesterol and high blood pressure, which explains why they are so effective at maintaining good brain health and even alleviating some of the symptoms of dementia. However, much of the research indicates that EPA and DHA have a slight edge over ALA. In light of this, it should come as no surprise to learn that marine food features prominently in the ManFood plan.

This is an important point to make, because it suggests that vegans and vegetarians may miss out on some of the protection that fish-eaters receive through their consumption of EPA and DHA, which are not found in plants. Therefore, this is one of the few occasions when supplementation may prove advantageous, because some of the omega 3 supplements that are specifically formulated for vegans and vegetarians are derived from marine algae and so contain EPA and DHA as well as ALA.

Antioxidants

Antioxidants are a group of nutrients that offer some protection against the damage caused by oxidative stress, which itself is a natural by-product of normal cell metabolism. The compounds that cause this damage, which are known as free radicals, have the potential to harm any cell, but they are especially detrimental to chemical structures with a double bond, such as 'good' fats. As the brain is largely composed of these fats, it is highly susceptible to free-radical damage.

Predictably, then, brain scans of people with Alzheimer's usually reveal evidence of the sort of lesions that are associated with free-radical exposure. Intriguingly, though, the same brains also tend to have higher than average levels of antioxidants and antioxidant activity, which perhaps suggests that the brain is trying its utmost to counteract the harmful effects of the free radicals.

Several nutrients have significant antioxidant potential, including vitamins C and E, selenium, copper, flavonoids, carotenoids and polyphenols. Some of these act on their own, while the body turns others into powerful antioxidant compounds. A complete list of all the foods that contain antioxidants would fill the rest of this book, but suffice it to say that they are found in the highest concentrations in fruits, vegetables, whole grains, nuts and seeds.

Yet again, I must stress that supplemented nutrients tend to be less effective than those that are ingested in food form, possibly because the supplements have been isolated from other compounds that may have some sort of synergistic influence. As always, think food first, not supplements.

Alcohol

The debate about whether alcohol is generally good or bad for our health rumbles on. However, in terms of dementia, the evidence is becoming increasingly irrefutable. In particular, excess or binge drinking seems to be a significant risk factor for developing the condition.

Historically, men have tended to drink more than women, perhaps in part because we have a slightly higher capacity for alcohol due to our larger livers. Nevertheless, since 2016, the guidelines have been the same for both sexes – a *maximum* of 14 units per week. (Previously, men were advised to drink no more than 21 units per week.) One unit is 10ml or 8g of pure alcohol, but this is not much help when you are trying to work out how much you can drink safely, given that the level of alcohol varies enormously depending on the type of drink.

You are probably familiar with the abbreviation 'ABV', which stands for 'alcohol by volume' – a measure of the amount of alcohol in a particular drink. New World wines (from South Africa, New Zealand and Australia) tend to be about 14 per cent ABV, whereas European wines are usually a percentage point or two lower. Traditional ales come in at about 3.5 per cent, but strong European beers and lagers may contain anything from 6 to 9 per cent. Therefore, it's hardly surprising that many people find it hard to keep track. A useful rule of thumb is that a large

(250ml) glass of wine or a pint of strong lager contains about 3 units. Meanwhile, a small (150ml) glass of wine or a pint of traditional draught ale contains roughly 2 units. Spirits, such as whisky, vodka and rum, are usually around 40 per cent ABV (although some brands can go as high as 57 per cent). A standard pub measure of average-strength vodka or whisky is about 35ml, which equates to 1.4 units.

Therefore, to keep within the official safe limits, you should allow yourself no more than six pints of beer, six modest glasses of wine or ten single measures of whisky each *week*. However, many people routinely exceed these amounts in a single *night*. And this isn't just a case of a group of rowdy youths on a pub crawl. Think of a sophisticated dinner party when your host greets you with a generous gin and tonic, followed by a couple of large glasses of wine during the meal, then a brandy with your coffee just before you leave. In the course of three or four seemingly very civilised hours, you have placed yourself in the category of binge drinker and exceeded your entire weekly allowance of alcohol.

This is important, because many studies have found that excessive alcohol consumption is a major risk factor for all types of dementia, especially early onset (under 65 years of age). And remember, what the scientists deem excessive tends to be far less than most people imagine.

A handful of studies have suggested that polyphenols, which are found in quite large quantities in red wine, might counteract the build-up of plaque in the brain. However, it should be pointed out that these chemicals are also found in tea, berries, kiwi fruit, cocoa and coffee. I guess the headline writers felt that 'Kiwi Stops Dementia' would sell fewer papers than 'Red Wine Halts Alzheimer's', so they decided to focus on the latter.

One final point to mention is that alcohol has exactly the same effect on the body – and particularly the brain – whether the source is an excellent Bordeaux consumed during a Michelin-starred meal or a bottle of strong cider swigged from a paper bag on a park bench. Persistent overindulgence of either will increase your risk of developing dementia later in life.

Sleep

Sleep is so crucial to general health and well-being that I have devoted the whole of the next chapter to the subject. Unsurprisingly, then, there is a well-established link between dementia and sleep disturbance, which tends to worsen as the condition progresses.

Some researchers have suggested that recurring problems in a particular phase of sleep might result in damage to the brain during what is commonly known as pre-dementia. On the other hand, it is possible that the damage occurs first and then disrupts the natural sleep cycle. It's a chicken and egg situation, and as yet no one has conclusively established whether sleep problems are one of the causes or one of the symptoms of dementia. All we do know is that the two tend to go hand in hand.

During healthy sleep, you pass through five distinct stages. One of these – rapid eye movement (REM) – occurs around ninety minutes after you fall asleep. All of the others are known collectively as non-rapid eye movement (NREM) stages. REM is categorised separately because the brain is especially active during this stage, probably because this is when we consolidate our memories. The first period of REM each night usually lasts no more than about ten minutes, but later episodes can continue for an hour or more before the mind moves on to the next NREM stage. Dreams are often extremely vivid during REM, as the brain can be just as active as it is during the day. By contrast, brain waves are much slower during the more sedate NREM phases.

We already know that alcohol consumption, both in excess

and late in the evening, can disturb REM. Moreover, some early research suggests that beta-amyloid – the main component of plaque – accumulates in the hippocampus when REM and NREM are disrupted. If true, this would certainly have a detrimental effect on the brain's ability to store new memories.

Mild cognitive impairment

Forgetting a name, or where you left your glasses, happens to all of us, especially as we get older. So there's no need to think that these increasingly regular occurrences indicate the onset of serious cognitive decline. On the other hand, if you start to experience significant changes in memory, judgement and/ or language, you may be in the early stages of 'mild cognitive impairment'.

It is almost impossible to define this condition with any sort of precision, but it is typified by forgetting events and appointments, an inability to follow the plot of a movie or a book, increasing impulsiveness, and problems with understanding simple instructions or advice. The brains of people living with mild cognitive impairment often have increased levels of plaque as well as a smaller than average hippocampus, due to shrinkage. And sufferers of the condition are at increased risk of developing dementia. Unsurprisingly, then, all of the aforementioned nutrients that can help in the fight against Alzheimer's and dementia may prove similarly effective against mild cognitive impairment.

Memory problems

Smoking, alcohol and illicit drugs can all have a detrimental effect on memory. For instance, long-term smoking tends to thin the cortex, the outer layer of the brain that plays an important role in various memory, language and perception functions. It should be said that a thinning cortex is a natural part of the ageing process, which may explain why we all find it more difficult to remember people's names or where we parked the car as we enter the latter stages of life, but the deterioration is much more pronounced in smokers.

As mentioned earlier, some forms of alcohol – most famously red wine – contain antioxidant and anti-inflammatory polyphenols and flavonoids that may offer some protection against Alzheimer's disease and dementia. However, exactly the same antioxidants are also found in grape juice and non-alcoholic beer, so you could get all of the benefits without ever exposing yourself to the harmful effects of alcohol.

If you think it's unrealistic to go entirely teetotal, the *amount* you drink is key. While three glasses of red wine a week may offer some protection to the hippocampus, routine consumption of more than that gradually reduces the brain's capacity to store new memories. Red wine's protective properties may be linked to the presence of a polyphenol called resveratrol, which is found in particularly high concentrations in Pinot Noir from cooler wine-growing regions, such as Bordeaux and Oregon. Once again, though, there are plenty of good non-alcoholic sources, including berries, cocoa and pistachio nuts.

A number of studies have found that resveratrol may slow cognitive decline. However, these trials have tended to test the effects of highly concentrated supplements, rather than resveratrol derived from dietary sources. Indeed, volunteers have usually been given levels that are equivalent to drinking 100 glasses of red wine each day! Obviously, the harmful effects of even a fiftieth of that amount of alcohol far outweigh any potential benefits. Therefore, as dull as it may sound, if you drink, try to keep your intake within the official guidelines.

Nutrients and cognitive function

If we were to compile a list of every dietary nutrient, it would be easier to highlight those that are *not* involved in some sort of brain function, rather than those that are. However, it is the antioxidants that play the most significant role in maintaining cognitive function. These include polyphenols, carotenoids, vitamins A, C and E, and the minerals selenium and zinc, most of which have anti-inflammatory properties too. As we have seen, omega 3 fats are also crucial, as is fibre, primarily because it can help to reduce cholesterol, so a balanced, healthy diet should include plenty of wholegrains, legumes and nuts. Finally, choline is involved in cell signalling and nerve transmission throughout the body, so an adequate supply is essential for the maintenance of cognitive function. Egg yolk, liver, peanuts, salmon, chickpeas, spinach, poultry and red meat are all particularly good sources.

As for what *not* to eat, the human body requires very little saturated fat to function correctly, while trans fats have no health benefits whatsoever. Therefore, both are best avoided as much as possible. You should also remain mindful about sugar and simple carbs, partly because they are broken down rapidly in the digestive system, leading to glucose spikes in the bloodstream, which in turn trigger the pancreas to release insulin. This is an entirely natural bodily process, but consistently high glucose levels may ultimately reduce the effectiveness of insulin and is a contributing factor in inflammation that will harm the brain as well as most other parts of the body.

In summary, we should all follow a diet that contains plenty of fruit, vegetables, wholegrains and fish, whereas we should limit our consumption of meat to maybe three or four meals a week, and certainly stick to the recommended guidelines with respect to alcohol.

CHAPTER 4

Sleep

It's more important than you might think

How much sleep do you get? How much do you need? Do we all need the same amount? And what happens if we don't get it?

Studies suggest that most adults need between seven and nine hours of sleep a night to maintain optimum health, although this falls to between five and seven hours over the age of 65. Personally, I tend to wake up around 6 a.m., and I'm usually ready for bed by 10 p.m. If I stay up beyond midnight, I know that I will struggle the next day, so I try to manage my diary to ensure that I'll be asleep (as opposed to merely in bed) by 10 p.m. the following evening. Friends and family sometimes tease me about this 'obsession' with getting a good night's sleep, but I know what I can manage and how ineffective I become whenever I fall out of my usual routine. Moreover, I have seen the harmful effects of long-term insomnia among many clients.

On average, it is estimated than men need about twenty minutes less sleep per night than women. However, we are all different. Consider Margaret Thatcher, who famously slept for only four hours a night throughout her premiership, or Winston Churchill, who took a lengthy nap every afternoon. Interestingly, both of these prime ministers behaved somewhat against their gender stereotypes, because sociology researchers at the University of Surrey found that men who boasted of needing only a few hours' sleep each night were considered 'macho', while oversleeping was viewed as self-indulgent or an indication that the person was struggling to keep up. Although the American Academy of Sleep Medicine acknowledges that we are all increasingly likely to suffer from insomnia as we age, it suggests that the condition is more prevalent among women. But could this be a simple case of women accepting that they have a problem and seeking help, whereas men ignore it, partly because they do not wish to appear unmanly? Certainly, men of my age were raised to 'get on with it' – feeling tired was *never* a valid excuse.

What you eat may not be the first thing that springs to mind when you think about sleep duration and quality, but several nutrients have a significant influence on both. We will explore these in detail later. First, though, we need to take a closer look at sleep itself.

What happens when you don't get enough sleep?

To some extent, sleeping – or at least sleeping for the recommended amount of time – can seem optional. Given the never-ending tasks that we all have to undertake in terms of earning a living, commuting, looking after the family, domestic chores, socialising, entertainment and exercise, achieving a minimum of seven hours of sleep every night might appear highly optimistic. Moreover, after meeting all of your commitments for the day, taking a little time to read a book or watch a movie may seem both well deserved and worthwhile. However, this sort of 'relaxation' often comes at the expense of sleep.

To examine whether this trade-off is worth it, we need to look at the functions of sleep, and explore why missing out may affect you now and in the future.

During non-REM sleep, the pituitary gland secretes human growth hormone (HGH), which plays a vital role in stimulating the repair and regrowth of tissue, muscle and bone throughout the body. Similarly, testosterone – which is linked to energy level, strength, libido and mood – is also secreted while we sleep, although in this instance primarily during the REM stage. A natural part of the ageing process is that production of both HGH and testosterone starts to decline as we enter middle age. However, in both cases, insufficient sleep may exacerbate the problem, which can lead to a noticeable deficiency of both hormones.

Two other hormones, leptin and ghrelin, are also affected by the amount of sleep. The former is released at the moment when your body decides you have eaten enough, quelling your appetite, whereas levels of the latter rise when your body needs fuel, causing you to experience hunger pangs. Unsurprisingly, leptin is secreted consistently while we sleep, signalling to the brain that no food is needed, while ghrelin levels fall. Therefore, insufficient sleep upsets the natural balance between the two hormones, making it more likely that you will feel hungry and overeat during waking hours.

The proper functioning of the immune system is also strongly associated with the amount of sleep we get. White blood cells known as T cells form part of our complex defence mechanism against threats such as pathogens and viruses, but the level of these crucial antibodies tends to fall when we are sleep deprived. T cells' specific role is to find and deactivate cells that have become infected, so lack of sleep is likely to have a detrimental effect on our ability to overcome disease. Meanwhile, the levels of inflammatory substances often increase when sleep is scarce.

As we saw in Chapter 3, age-related changes to the brain also seem to be exacerbated by a lack of sleep. The brain processes the events of the previous day while we sleep, essentially discarding the unimportant details while committing the more significant events to memory. Obviously, this process is impaired when sleep is insufficient or interrupted.

Finally, there's cortisol. Production of this hormone is usually highest first thing in the morning, then gradually declines as the day progresses, falling to its lowest level when the body recognises that it is time to sleep. It plays a crucial role in making glucose available to meet the body's routine energy requirements, but it is secreted in particularly large quantities at times of stress (which could be anything from running for a bus to suffering a bereavement). Its principal function is to increase blood pressure, which enables the rapid transport of glucose and other nutrients to where they are most needed during a crisis. However, if the stress continues and cortisol levels remain unnaturally high until late in the evening, it can be very difficult to fall asleep, or indeed remain asleep throughout the night. Moreover, raised cortisol levels one night often lead to an even greater elevation the following night, resulting in a vicious circle.

Foods that aid sleep

A number of dietary nutrients can improve both the quality and duration of sleep, but their effect is generally cumulative and gentle, rather than immediate and intense, as is the case with sleeping pills and indeed a couple of supplements.

Vitamin D

At present, the precise mechanism by which vitamin D affects sleep is uncertain, but many studies have reached the same conclusion: namely, that low levels of this vitamin are associated with both insomnia and poor-quality sleep.

As we saw in Chapter 2, vitamin D is produced by the skin during exposure to sunlight, and it is also found in various foods, such as oily fish, portobello mushrooms and egg yolks. However, this is one of those rare instances when the best way to ensure a consistent supply is to take a supplement.

Magnesium

Magnesium promotes healthy sleep because, in addition to encouraging muscle relaxation, it is a key component of a neurotransmitter that carries messages from the brain to the central nervous system. The full name of this neurotransmitter is gamma-aminobutyric acid, but it is usually known as GABA. It has a mild sedative effect and so helps to offset the symptoms of anxiety and stress, including insomnia.

Foods that are particularly rich in magnesium include pumpkin seeds, spinach, oats, brown rice, quinoa, nuts and lentils, but any green vegetable will do as they all get their distinctive colour from chlorophyll, which itself is a good source of magnesium.

I sometimes advise clients to take a magnesium supplement if they are struggling to sleep. These usually come in 100mg or 200mg tablets, and most people find that a dose of 200mg is helpful. A word of warning, however: magnesium also has a laxative effective, so use it with caution.

Indeed, rather than running headlong down the supplement path, try keeping a sleep diary for a week or two first. Each morning, record how easily you fell asleep the night before and whether you enjoyed a restful night's sleep. If this reveals a recurring problem, try a 100mg dose of magnesium half an hour before going to bed for a few nights, then gradually build up to

200mg, if necessary. Continue to record the results in your sleep diary and monitor your progress.

A SLEEP DIARY

My sleep diary includes four main categories:

- How alert do I feel?
- How tired do I feel?
- Do I feel focused?
- How well did I sleep last night?

I then rate each of these on a scale of 1 to 10. So, for instance, 1 would signify 'completely exhausted', while 10 would equate to 'boundless energy'. Of course, you can tailor these categories to the feelings and sensations that are most important and relevant to you. In addition, you should note factors such as level of stress, alcohol and caffeine consumption, and duration and periods of screen use.

Keeping a record of your scores over two weeks will help you to establish whether your sleep problems are linked to lifestyle. If you decide that they are, you can start to make the necessary adjustments, but remember to continue with the diary, as this will reveal which changes are having the most positive effects.

Vitamin B1

Vitamin B1 (otherwise known as thiamine) is also involved in the production of GABA, so, predictably, any deficiency of the vitamin can result in low levels of the neurotransmitter. It is found in wholegrains, lentils, black beans, barley, green peas, oats and pork, but sunflower seeds are the best source.

Melatonin

The hormone melatonin, which is secreted by the pineal gland in the very centre of the brain, is directly related to sleep. Production automatically increases as daylight starts to fade, inducing sleepiness, and decreases at dawn, causing us to wake. However, our capacity to manufacture melatonin starts to decline as we age, which is one reason why insomnia becomes more of an issue for many people later in life.

Bearing in mind that melatonin production decreases whenever the body senses light, staring at a laptop, tablet or smartphone late in the evening keeps levels of melatonin unnaturally low at the very moment when they should be on the rise. Therefore, it's a good idea to turn off every screen at least an hour and a half before you intend to fall asleep, as this should give your melatonin levels a chance to build up.

Melatonin occurs naturally in walnuts, mustard seeds, ginger, peanuts and oats, although tart cherries are possibly the best dietary source, especially when juiced. Some small-scale studies into age-related insomnia have found that drinking a shot of tart cherry juice increases melatonin levels, and participants reported both longer and better sleep. Therefore, it may be worth experimenting with a shot of cherry juice each night for a week if you are having trouble falling asleep or find yourself waking up in the middle of the night. It is widely available in health-food stores. If you try this then do so without taking magnesium, so that you can better assess the outcome of taking the supplement.

Valerian and hops

Alternative and traditional medicine practitioners often prescribe the root of the valerian plant as a sedative. However, the scientific studies into its effectiveness are far from conclusive, with many trials reporting little or no benefit. On the other hand, some researchers have suggested that long-term use may increase the duration of deep sleep. If so, this may be because valerian boosts the action of GABA.

From personal experience, it seems that valerian tea might at least speed up the process of falling asleep. I leave a teabag to steep in hot water for ten minutes, then drink the tea half an hour before getting into bed. It works for me, and a number of clients have reported positive results too, but these experiments should not be considered robust scientific research. In addition, you should bear in mind that any soporific effect can continue into the next day, so take care if you decide to give valerian a try.

Some brands of valerian tea also contain hops, which are said to have a similar effect. The two can also be found in herbal tinctures. A few drops, added to hot water, can be just as effective as steeping a teabag for ten minutes, but you must be careful not to exceed the recommended dose, as this can induce daytime drowsiness.

Carbohydrates

Eating a carb-rich meal, as opposed to a protein-rich meal, a couple of hours before going to bed may encourage sleep. This is because protein-rich meals contain countless different types of amino acids, all of which compete with each other to cross the semi-permeable membrane that separates the bloodstream from the brain. By contrast, carb-rich meals contain far fewer amino acids, which allows one particular type – tryptophan – to enter the brain without hindrance. Once there, it boosts the production of the main sleep hormone, melatonin.

Therefore, if you have trouble falling asleep, you might think that it's a good idea to eat lots of carbs every evening. Unfortunately, though, overcoming insomnia is not that easy, because a high-carb meal may also result in a spike in blood glucose, potentially resulting in a burst of energy that could far exceed the soporific effect of the tryptophan.

There's no easy solution to this paradox, although I certainly would not advocate eating only protein and vegetables after 6 p.m., as several weight-loss plans suggest. In addition to reducing the beneficial effect of tryptophan, such an approach is simply impractical for most people.

Foods that hinder sleep

Caffeine

About a decade ago, during an especially stressful life episode, I decided to cut out all caffeine, as I felt that it was adding to my anxiety. It was far easier than I expected, and I decided to continue with decaffeinated coffee once my life returned to normal. Last year, though, I decided to reintroduce caffeine, and now I enjoy the slight lift it gives me first thing in the morning.

Caffeine is much maligned in some quarters, but there is nothing wrong with it as long as it is ingested in small quantities, especially as most of us consume it in the forms of tea and coffee, both of which are excellent sources of various antioxidants, including polyphenols. It has a similar chemical structure to adenosine, a neurotransmitter that encourages sleep, so part of its stimulant effect is due to the fact that it blocks some of the adenosine receptors in the brain. In turn, this triggers the adrenal glands to produce adrenaline and cortisol, two stress hormones that make us feel more alert. It can take up to forty-five minutes for coffee to work its magic, but thereafter the effect can last for four hours.

The problems begin when we have too much. If the adenosine receptors are repeatedly blocked by excessive consumption of caffeine, the brain responds by making more. Over time, this can mean that you need to drink coffee not to get the benefit of increased alertness but merely to stop feeling tired. The problem is that a breakfast coffee seems to be an easy way to get a quick energy boost after a poor night's sleep, but that poor night's sleep might be due, at least in part, to the caffeine you drank the previous day. Therefore, it can fast become a vicious circle.

It is estimated that 10 per cent of adults metabolise caffeine quickly and have a naturally high tolerance for it. These people can consume it late in the day without affecting their sleep patterns. For the rest of us, however, while caffeine may provide a temporary lift, increased tolerance is often associated with anxiety, stress and insomnia.

Caffeine is found in cocoa as well as tea and coffee, although the amount depends on how the beans are processed. In general, however, the caffeine in a product increases in line with the amount of cocoa it contains, so 50g of dark chocolate (70 per cent cocoa) may contain as much as 50mg of caffeine – roughly equivalent to a single espresso. Colas contain plenty of caffeine, too, with a can of regular Coke having around 34mg and the diet version 45mg. Compare these amounts to the 60mg you will get from one coffee pod or the 80–115mg in a cup of strong brewed coffee. A mug of tea contains around 75mg, while a large cup of instant coffee provides 100mg. Given these figures, it is easy to see why so many people far exceed the recommended 400mg of caffeine each day.

If you are suffering from insomnia, my advice is to eliminate all caffeine from your diet for a couple of weeks and record any changes in the duration and quality of your sleep. Then you can start to reintroduce *modest* amounts of caffeine and will be able to assess how much you can tolerate before the problems start to recur.

Alcohol

While most of us are aware that a double espresso is not the best idea just before we turn in for the night, few people realise that alcohol can be similarly detrimental to a good night's sleep. I was teetotal for a number of years and now just have the occasional glass of wine with dinner. Nevertheless, even that modest amount can sometimes be enough to leave me feeling that I'm not firing on all cylinders the next day. Then, needless to say, the knee-jerk reaction is to reach for the caffeine. Before long, you can fall into an unhelpful caffeine–alcohol–caffeine loop.

The body responds to alcohol by secreting more adenosine, which promotes relaxation and sleepiness, so a few late-night drinks can certainly help you fall asleep. Unfortunately, the problems begin a few hours later. Under normal circumstances, levels of adenosine decline naturally and gradually throughout the night. However, when production has been boosted by alcohol, they can fall much more rapidly. This may lead to seemingly inexplicable waking in the middle of the night and hinder your ability to get back to sleep. In addition, even if you remain asleep for seven or eight hours after drinking alcohol, you are likely to experience much less REM sleep than usual, which can have a profound impact on both mood and energy levels the next day.

Once again, if you suffer from night-time waking or other sleep problems that you suspect may be alcohol-related, the best idea is to keep a sleep diary. This will reveal any link between the two and then you can take the necessary action, such as limiting or even eliminating your consumption of alcohol in the evening.

CHAPTER 5

Managing your weight

It's about more than simple aesthetics

Weight issues are probably the most debated topic among the nutritional community, and everyone has an opinion. Unfortunately, though, information from professional nutritionists, which is based on attainment of the appropriate qualifications, years of study and clinical experience and a deep understanding of the subject, is all too often drowned out by the ill-informed theories of television presenters, celebrities and personal trainers. These contributions have tended to make an already emotive topic more confusing than it should be.

Although the diet industry has traditionally focused most of its attention on the female population, men are far from immune to weight gain. Indeed, 68 per cent of adult men in the UK are considered overweight or obese, compared to 58 per cent of women. Nor are we immune to countless theories regarding how to lose some of that excess weight. However, most male weight-loss plans tend to concentrate on exercise, at the expense of diet. While good health is usually linked to slimness among women, for men it's usually associated with fitness and rippling muscles. All too often, the idea seems to be that you can eat whatever you want, as long as you put in enough hours down the gym or pounding the streets. In theory that may be true but you'd have to work very hard and never miss a day to make it so. I believe that roughly 80 per cent of weight gain (and consequently weight loss) is due to diet, while exercise accounts for only 20 per cent. To put it simply, you can't outrun a bad diet; it will always catch up with you before too long.

That said, it's undoubtedly important to remain active as you age, in part to maintain muscle mass. Interestingly, men have a slight natural advantage over women when it comes to weight loss because, on average, we have larger muscles, which means we have more potential to turn stored fat into energy. However, muscle mass starts to decline as a natural part of the ageing process from around the age of 30 onwards, so it's a good idea to counteract this with some weight-training. You don't have to become a body-builder – just incorporate some mild strengthening exercises into your routine a few times each week.

In addition, you might want to consider employing a personal trainer, if only for a couple of sessions to set you on the right path (but note that it should be for advice on exercise, and not also on nutrition, as many have only a rudimentary training in this complex area). You might already play tennis, squash or football, too. If so, that's great, but it's also advisable to think about how active (or otherwise) you are when you're *not* on the pitch or at the gym. Let's say you exercise two or three times each week. That probably amounts to no more than 3 or 4 out of a total of 112 waking hours (assuming you get 8 hours' sleep a night). Ideally, you should incorporate some sort of physical activity within the other 100-plus hours, such as walking, stretching or just moving whenever you can. Perhaps you could follow the 10,000 steps per day programme? Or possibly take the stairs rather than the lift?

Eventually, though, there will probably come a time when you won't be able to exercise at the same level, or possibly even at all. That's why it's imperative to pay attention to diet as well as exercise. In terms of health, and to help you lose weight, they go together like chips and ketchup, or should that be quinoa and kale?

ARE YOU OVERWEIGHT?

You can work out your Body Mass Index, or BMI, by dividing your weight in kilos by your height in metres squared. So, if you are 1.8 metres tall and weigh 80 kilos, your BMI is:

$$80 \div 1.8^2 = 24.7$$

A BMI of 18.5 is considered 'underweight'; anything between 18.6 and 24.9 is classified as 'normal'; 25–29.9 is 'overweight'; and over 30 is deemed 'obese'.

However, in practice, BMI is quite a blunt instrument as it doesn't distinguish between fat and muscle, so a top-class athlete may have exactly the same BMI as an inactive couch potato. For this reason, many people now prefer to use a simple piece of string to determine if they are overweight.

Measure out a piece of string to match your height, cut it in half, then try to circle your waist with one of the halves. If you can get it around your midriff easily, then your amount of visceral fat (that is, all of the fat throughout your body, not just in your belly) is acceptable. On the other hand, if you struggle to make the two ends meet, your level of visceral fat is probably too high.

Why you should lose excess weight

Excess weight is linked to many of the health issues that are discussed throughout this book. For example, hypertension is twice as likely to affect an overweight or obese man than a man with normal BMI. To put it another way, carrying more fat than you should means you have a 43 per cent chance of developing high blood pressure.

Cholesterol is also likely to be raised if you are overweight, as are blood glucose levels. We know that excess weight is a significant risk factor in developing type 2 diabetes as well as some forms of cancer, including colon and kidney cancer, and there is some evidence that the risk of pancreatic cancer is raised, too. In addition, partly because there is more weight for the joints to support, arthritis and other forms of joint pain are likely. Gout is also more common in men who need to lose weight.

Therefore, if you are carrying some extra weight, you should think about addressing the problem sooner rather than later.

Which factors influence our weight?

Over the last half-century or so, what we weigh has come to be the principal marker for health. If you are overweight, you are considered unhealthy, regardless of the quality of your diet. Nevertheless, older men, by which I mean those in middle age and above, are less likely than any other group to lose weight, or even acknowledge that they need to.

Muscle versus fat

Some weight gain is viewed as inevitable as the years pass, and to some extent this is true. As mentioned above, we all start to lose muscle mass as we age, with inactive men over the age of 30 losing between 2 and 5 per cent each decade. More active men may delay this process, but even they will generally start to lose some muscle mass by their late forties. In turn, there tends to be a corresponding increase in the amount of fat in our bodies.

This is important, because muscle is far more efficient than fat in terms of using the energy that is generated from the food you eat. I should add that when I speak of 'muscle', I don't necessarily mean huge biceps and a well-defined six-pack. All of us have muscles throughout our bodies and they all burn energy – it's just the size that varies.

Hormones

Another factor in age-related weight gain is the gradual decline in testosterone levels. These peak during puberty and young adulthood, plateau for a few years, then start to decrease by about 1 per cent per year from the age of 30 onwards. Testosterone plays an important role in protein synthesis and also encourages the production of growth hormones – two factors that are related to maintaining and building muscle mass. In addition, as levels fall, fat storage tends to increase. This may lead you to believe that taking testosterone supplements is an easy means to combat weight gain and loss of muscle, but this can have serious side-effects and there are many other factors to consider, too. Therefore, you should always consult your doctor before deciding to embark on this course of action (see Chapter 8 for more details).

Insulin is also an important factor in weight gain, especially as we get older. It is produced in the pancreas in response to rising blood glucose levels after eating and drinking, whereupon it encourages the movement of the glucose into cells, where it is used to make energy. It can also shunt away glucose that is surplus to requirements, preserving it for later use (see Chapter 7 for more details).

There are also the two appetite-control hormones that we

met earlier – leptin and ghrelin. The former, which is secreted from several parts of the body, mostly by fat cells, switches off the hunger response. Therefore, people who are overweight tend to have higher levels of leptin than those who are underweight, as their large numbers of fat cells try to tell them to stop eating. However, over time, the body becomes desensitised to leptin and its signals are no longer acknowledged. Consequently, you can feel ravenous even when you have had more than enough to eat.

Ghrelin has the opposite effect to leptin. Produced by specific cells in the stomach and the pancreas, it sends hunger signals to the brain. Hence, levels increase before a meal, and then *should* decline after eating. However, as we saw in Chapter 4, this natural rise and fall can be thrown out of balance by other factors, such as lack of sleep.

The microbiome

The trillions of bacteria that reside primarily in our intestines can also influence our weight. Collectively known as the microbiome, each of us has a unique combination of bacteria that affects how the body processes the carbohydrates, protein and fat we eat.

Trials have found that swapping the microbiome of a rat that gains weight easily with one that eats the same amount yet maintains a healthy weight reverses the situation. You may well find the notion of a fecal transplant repugnant, but it's interesting to note that simply maintaining good gut health can help weight management. (I discuss this in more depth in Chapter 10.) Nevertheless, calories still count, even for those with the healthiest microbiomes.

Family history

Genetics can have a profound influence on our ability to process carbohydrates, fat and protein, and therefore on our susceptibility to gain weight. However, family history involves more than just the genes we inherit from our parents.

You should also consider the role that food and diets have played in your home life ever since childhood. Perhaps certain members of your family have been in a never-ending cycle of dieting, then lapsing back into bad habits, then dieting again. In the 1970s and 1980s, their diets of choice were probably low-fat plans. Later, the focus shifted to fibre, then fat, then protein. Diets are constantly falling in and out of fashion, but even if you've never tried one yourself, and are quite sceptical about the whole 'diet industry', the chances are that they have had some impact on how you think about food. In addition, during childhood, you were probably bribed to eat your greens with the promise of dessert, and you may have witnessed others being judged as 'good' or 'bad', depending on whether they were thin or fat. These early experiences should not be underestimated, as they stay with us and can have long-lasting impacts on how we feel about food, treats, indulgence and how to lose weight.

If these cumulative experiences have led you to believe that weight loss is always difficult, and that any excess pounds you have gained are all your own fault, then you probably also believe that you deserve to suffer the 'punishment' of an arduous diet and exercise regime.

This perception of weight – fat is always bad, slim is always good – pervades the language of almost every diet plan, but it can be anything but healthy over the long term. Therefore, if you have found yourself uttering any of the following phrases, you may need to readjust your thinking on diets and weight loss:

- I've been so good
- I've slipped up
- I've been bad all weekend
- I'll start afresh on Monday
- Go on, you're on holiday/it's your birthday
- I deserve it because I've done so well all week
- I feel so guilty
- A couple of mouthfuls won't hurt
- OK, I will, but just to be polite

Of course, some of these expressions may be valid at certain times, but they all reinforce the notion that food is generally bad – something to be feared or shunned, rather than enjoyed. They encourage a feast-or-famine mindset rather than moderation, and ignore meaningful nutrition, instead focusing simply on whether certain foods will make you fat or thin.

How to diet successfully

In the twenty years since I started in nutritional practice, I have seen countless diets come and go. The normal chain of events is that a supposedly revolutionary approach is published in a high-profile book and the author then embarks on a round of interviews with magazines, newspapers, TV and radio, during which, ideally, they will drop the names of a few celebrities who have achieved remarkable results by following the diet. In addition, the health markers that accompany all weight loss – such as increased energy and better blood test results – are discussed as if they are unique to this specific diet. Ultimately, the author achieves a degree of fame and 'expert' status, and the media continues to seek their opinion on subsequent weight-loss plans and all other aspects of nutrition. They may well advocate a particular 'food philosophy' that defines what they themselves eat, and they might be fortunate enough to reap the benefits of follow-up books, updated diet plans or even a TV series with a celebrity chef as co-host. However, they need to strike while the iron is hot, because another diet will soon become flavour of the month.

To some extent, I am writing from personal experience here, as I published one or two diet books in the mid-2000s that resulted in a level of visibility I never would have achieved if I had focused on any other aspect of health. However, what I wrote then remains as valid as ever, not because it was unique, not because I had discovered some weight-loss secret that had previously been overlooked or misunderstood (two time-honoured ways to publicise diet books), but because the plan was practical and addressed wider nutritional requirements. It also worked *with* natural bodily functions, not against them.

You have probably seen numerous stories of people who have lost weight by following a specific plan and report lower blood pressure, reduced cholesterol, more energy, better sleep and so on. The implication is that all of these benefits are due to the particular approach that was followed, but in reality they are much more likely to be natural consequences of the weight loss itself, not the diet that was used to achieve it.

So, is there some kind of common denominator among all of the popular diets? Well, yes there is. No matter how they get there – by reducing fat, increasing fat, bulking up on fibre, or whatever – the ultimate aim of every weight-loss plan is simply to reduce the total intake of calories. Of course, the better ones aim to provide some additional benefits, such as improved gut health or increased muscle mass. However, in order to lose weight, there is no way round the fact that your body has to be placed in energy deficit.

Just as body fat is essentially a storage facility for all of the food you eat that is surplus to your energy requirements, you must eat less to create an energy shortfall and force those fat cells to release their contents.

It really is the only way.

If a diet drastically reduces your calories, it *will* work. You *will* lose weight. But is it practical? Is it sustainable over the long term? Is it affordable? Does it fit in with your lifestyle, commitments and obligations? Does it address wider nutritional needs?

CALORIES

Not all foodstuffs contain the same amount of calories. Protein and carbohydrates both contain 4 calories per gram, whereas fat contains 9. The high calorific content of fat is the reason why so many diets of the 1970s and 1980s were either fat-free or low-fat, because avoiding fat almost guaranteed an overall reduction in calories. However, cutting out all fat can have some unfortunate consequences, such as eliminating hugely beneficial omega 3 fats from the diet.

Current guidelines suggest that an adult male needs no more than 2500 calories a day, although this figure is an average and may vary depending on age, certain medical issues and levels of particular hormones. Hence, some men might need only 2000, while others could eat more and not gain weight. For example, a man in his mid-sixties would generally need only 2200 calories to remain healthy.

Personally, I aim to eat a 500-calorie breakfast, 700 calories at both lunch and dinner, and 300 calories in mid-morning and mid-afternoon snacks, all of which adds up to the recommended 2500 calories for a man of my age. I find that this approach keeps my energy levels well balanced and my hunger manageable throughout the day, but it is not set in stone. I know many men who prefer to eat three larger meals a day, with no snacks in between. Remember, we are all different. You just have to find the best way to keep your consumption of calories within healthy limits.

Back in the 1970s, we all thought that it was fat in the diet that was making us fat. By 2000, the focus had shifted to carbs. Now, most of the blame is directed at sugar. But there's no point trying to identify a single culprit.

You put on weight simply by eating more than you need.

With that undeniable truth in mind, how do you choose the weight-loss plan that is best for you from the plethora of options that jostle for attention in bookstores, online forums and village halls and recreation centres up and down the country? And how do you ensure that it will meet your wider nutritional needs?

The Four Ps

If all weight-loss plans merely reduce your intake of calories, why not just go into a bookshop, randomly pick a diet book off the shelf and follow it?

Well, you probably could do that ... if you were bothered about nothing other than losing weight. But the ManFood approach considers much more besides. Its aim is to optimise your weight while also keeping you well supplied with all of the nutrients your body needs to maintain good health into middle age and beyond.

With this in mind, there is a checklist of issues to consider before embarking on any diet. I call these the Four Ps:

1. Practicality
- Does the diet plan suit your lifestyle, commitments and obligations? If it restricts you too much, or means that you cannot participate in activities you enjoy, or requires you to prepare food at home when time is scarce, is it really for you?
- How sustainable is it? Of course, you will lose weight if you reduce your intake of calories at first, but if you lapse later, what is the point? You will regain all the weight you lost, and may carry the added burden of feeling like a failure.

2. Price
- Any diet plan that far exceeds your budget will be unsustainable over the long term.
- Admittedly, some healthy food choices may cost a little more than burgers and buckets of fried chicken, but you don't need to spend a fortune on specialist ingredients in order to lose weight. Indeed, many of the foods that feature prominently in the ManFood plan – such as seasonal fresh fruit and vegetables – are anything but expensive.

3. Pleasure
- You are probably lucky enough to have access to a wide variety of delicious food. That means, if you are in your mid-fifties, you probably can look forward to another 35,000 meals. And you should look forward to them, because enjoying what you eat is a welcome component of any healthy diet.
- In addition, many people experience hunger in a very unsettling way, often engaging in a perpetual internal dialogue over whether they should give in to temptation or stay strong and resist. Many diets actively encourage

this sort of negative and masochistic mindset. Instead, you should choose one that promotes positivity and pleasure, rather than guilt.

4. Persistence
- Managing your weight is like looking after your finances: it's not something you need to do every now and again; it requires regular attention. Therefore, your diet plan should be sustainable and prudent, not boom and bust.
- Once you have reached a weight where you feel comfortable, and which puts you in the 'healthy' category across a range of markers (e.g. BMI between 18.5 and 25), you should aim to stay there.
- Obviously, you might gain a little during holidays or festivities, but if that happens you should address it as soon as the party is over and get back down to your optimum weight.

Common dieting pitfalls

In addition to what you eat, you should be aware of some other issues before embarking on a weight-loss diet:

1. Weekdays and weekends
- After following a strict routine during the week, it is all too easy to overindulge at the weekend, because you feel you deserve it, you've worked hard all week, it would be rude not to, etc.
- Unfortunately, though, in addition to guaranteeing a succession of miserable Monday mornings, going from feast to famine and back again is likely to halt your weight loss in its tracks.

- So-called 'cheat days', which many weight-loss plans now advocate (or at least tolerate), can often scupper a diet, too. Consistency is one of the keys to gradual, significant, healthy weight loss, so don't build in a day when you definitely cheat, rather allow it here and there.

2. Drinks and liquids
- What you drink can have an enormous impact on your calorie intake without you even noticing.
- Homemade tea and coffee contain minimal calories – maybe just 2 per mug – but a dash of milk can add 25, and a teaspoon of sugar a further 16.
- Meanwhile, coffees from high-street chains often have far more calories than you would imagine. For instance, a small latte made with whole milk comes in at 180 – or 108 for skimmed milk – while a grande provides 280 or 128, respectively. A cappuccino contains less milk, so a tall cup has 163 or 93 calories, respectively. So, let's say you have one cup of tea at home and a couple of cappuccinos during the day: that's a minimum of 250 calories. Of course, that's fine, as it's only a tenth of your recommended daily allowance. Just be aware of it.
- Alcohol is another matter entirely because, at 7 calories per gram, it's very easy to rack them up.
- The stronger the drink (i.e. the higher the ABV), the more calories it contains. A 250ml glass of medium-strength (13 per cent ABV) red or white wine provides 228 calories, while a 175ml glass has 160. Meanwhile, a pint of lager contains 180 calories, while a pint of beer has slightly more – 215. Prefer a gin and tonic? A single comes in at 97 calories, while a double has 149 (roughly equivalent to six squares of milk chocolate or five teaspoons of peanut butter).

3. Sleep, stress and hunger

- One of the many unwelcome side-effects of insomnia is increased hunger due to raised levels of the hormone ghrelin and a consequent tendency to snack more. This is entirely understandable as carbs, sugar and caffeine all have the potential to mitigate fatigue, but increasing your intake of calories in this way will make it very difficult to lose weight.

- Similarly, long-term stress leads to elevated levels of cortisol, which increases appetite in general, and cravings for fat and sugar in particular. After all, when have you ever seen someone reach for the broccoli when they are stressed?

4. Other people

- If you told a friend or relative that you were following the ManFood plan to reduce your risk of prostate enlargement or to combat your hypertension, they would almost certainly offer enthusiastic encouragement and support. The chances are that they would never even think of arguing with your decision or suggesting an alternative based on their own personal experience.

- However, if you tell someone your intention is to lose weight, you will usually find that everyone's an expert and has an opinion about what you should be doing. They may have your best interests at heart, but you must stick to your guns and do it your way.

Which diet is right for you?

So, how do you choose a diet that allows you to address the Four Ps while simultaneously avoiding all of the common dieting pitfalls? The most important point to remember is that, while all weight-loss plans rely on calorie deficit, you should never sacrifice your nutritional requirements in order to achieve this. You will be eating less, but you still need to ensure that you get all the nutrients you need.

A huge variety of options are available (see below for some of the most popular), and any one of them will help you lose excess weight, as long as you follow the plan correctly. As you will see, I do not recommend one in particular, as they all have their individual merits and drawbacks. Rather, I advise using the Four Ps as a checklist to guide you to whichever approach best suits your lifestyle and personal preferences. Regardless of which plan you choose, however, make sure that it corresponds with the basic principles of the ManFood plan, which are outlined in Part Two of this book.

Fasting diets

Fasting diets have become particularly popular over the last couple of years. Some advocate sticking to just 600 calories for two days a week, while others are based on eating for only eight hours, then fasting for sixteen (say, from eight-thirty in the evening to lunchtime the following afternoon) each day. Both of these approaches aid weight loss as you are guaranteed to eat less if you follow them correctly. Despite what some people think, you don't go mad by gorging on doughnuts and cheese when you are not in a fasting period.

I have found that fasting tends to suit people who prefer a strict plan with rules that they can follow. Much of the choice that is present in other approaches is eliminated – simply because there are fewer opportunities to eat during the day – and it often promotes a sense of satisfaction and achievement as the fasting periods become easier to tolerate.

However, it is not for everyone, as some people experience hunger and low energy far more keenly than others. Similarly, your work or other commitments may make it difficult to stick to a strict schedule of when you can and cannot eat, especially if you feel you need a boost of energy at precisely those moments when food is off the table.

Little and often

Eating small amounts of food at regular intervals is another good way to lose weight, especially if you suffer frequent hunger pangs and lack energy. This approach often suits people who work in offices or in places where there is easy access to a kitchen and/ or food outlets. It works as a weight-loss programme because it promotes a consistent level of glucose in the bloodstream, which is harder to achieve if you have three large meals per day. As we feel hunger when glucose levels are low – and convert excess glucose into fat – it makes sense to keep them as stable as possible.

Combining the main food groups – carbohydrates, protein and fat – can also help to maintain balanced blood sugar, as protein and particularly fat are digested relatively slowly. By contrast, carbohydrates – and especially simple carbs, such as those that are found white bread and pasta, fruit juices and sugar – are broken down very easily and quickly. In addition, most or all of the fibre is removed from these sorts of processed carbohydrates, which speeds up their conversion into glucose, boosting levels in the bloodstream. Compare, say, drinking the juice of an apple to eating the whole apple. The natural sugars are bound to fibre in the apple, which means the digestive system has to work hard to release them and convert them into glucose. By contrast, this process is much easier and quicker after drinking virtually fibre-free juice.

Therefore, the healthiest approach is to eat a combination of complex, fibrous carbs, protein and a little fat at every meal and snack. In simple terms, this will result in a gentle drip feed of glucose into the bloodstream, which in turn will mean that insulin, leptin and ghrelin are all kept in check.

Once you understand the principle, the practice is quite straightforward. For instance, you could add some walnuts to cereal to increase the levels of both fibre and fat in your breakfast. Or how about peanut butter, ham or smoked salmon on toast, rather than jam? An apple plus some hummus or pumpkin seeds makes a healthy snack, while dinner could be chicken or beans with rice and vegetables. It's always a good idea to ask 'Where's the protein?' every time you eat, and add some if it's missing.

Following this approach throughout the day should give you consistent energy while also keeping hunger pangs at bay and may work well for someone who struggles with hunger. If you do it right, you should start to feel moderately hungry just before each meal or snack, which will encourage you to satisfy your hunger but not overeat or make poor food choices.

High-protein diets

This approach advocates a high intake of protein, which is mostly eaten with green vegetables and a small amount of fat. Meanwhile, all carbs, and especially grains, fruits, starchy vegetables and beans, are strictly limited.

As protein takes much longer to digest than carbohydrates, it satisfies appetite for longer, so people on high-protein diets can eat less without feeling hungry, resulting in a calorie deficit and therefore weight loss. This type of diet also keeps insulin levels low and encourages the body to get its energy from compounds called ketones rather than its usual fuel, glucose. The body manufactures these from its reserves of stored fat whenever glucose is in short supply, as it is sure to be on a low-carb diet.

A typical daily menu might comprise Greek yoghurt with a few blueberries and nuts for breakfast, chicken with salad and crunchy green vegetables for lunch, and a dinner of steak with vegetables. Depending on the plan, you might be allowed a small portion of carbs – say, a tablespoon of brown rice or pasta – with lunch or dinner.

A word of warning: as the kidneys are involved in the final stages of protein metabolism, the high-protein approach is not recommended for anyone with renal damage, and it also increases the risk of developing kidney stones.

Low-carb, high-fat diets

Although this type of diet also incorporates a fair amount of protein, it differs from the previous approach because it includes far more fat and even fewer carbs. This means it is even more likely to encourage the body to run on ketones – a physical state known as ketosis – so it is sometimes termed the 'ketogenic' or 'keto' diet.

A typical breakfast might be cheese and nuts, or eggs cooked in coconut oil with sliced avocado, followed by salmon, more avocado and green vegetables with a sprinkling of seeds or nuts for lunch, and a dinner of chicken breast or steak with cheese sauce accompanied by green vegetables. Some of these plans also recommend adding coconut oil or even butter to coffee in order to boost the intake of fat and accelerate the body's entry into ketosis.

Remember, both fat and protein are much more satisfying than carbs, so keto diets are particularly good at mitigating hunger.

However, they are controversial, to say the least. Supporters are adamant that they are the only way to guarantee weight loss, whereas the majority of the established medical community largely dismiss them as misguided and faddy. Personally, I feel that, while a keto diet will almost certainly enable you to lose weight in a relatively short period of time, which will provide some health benefits, it will also deprive you of some of the essential nutrients you need to maintain general good health, such as carotenoids and flavanols. In addition, it can be very difficult to eat sufficient fibre on high-protein and especially keto plans, which can have serious consequences further down the line.

In my experience, both of these approaches are particularly attractive to men, perhaps because eating meat twice a day is seen as macho. Or maybe it's just that they are relatively easy to follow because hunger is minimised and many of the dishes are very flavourful. Indeed, given the high fat and protein content, it can scarcely feel like dieting at all. Nevertheless, because of the serious drawbacks with respect to nutrient and fibre deficiency, I would not recommend either of them over the long term.

Very low-calorie diets and meal replacements

As I have mentioned several times in this chapter, *all* diets cut calories in one way or another. However, some plans specifically highlight their low-calorie credentials. Typically, these approaches replace regular meals with specially prepared soups, smoothies or ready-meals that are low in calories because they contain either very little fat or none whatsoever.

This may sound like a good idea, given that a gram of fat contains more than twice as many calories as a gram of carbohydrate. However, as we learned earlier, fat is much more effective at satisfying hunger, so following one of these plans invariably demands a great deal of willpower. Of course, you may feel that you are blessed with an iron will and that enduring almost constant hunger is worth the sacrifice if it results in significant weight loss. Nevertheless, I don't believe that such diets are either sustainable or enjoyable, and they certainly do not offer the optimum nutrition that you require to maintain good health over the long term.

So, what is the answer?

Any one of the aforementioned diets will certainly help you lose weight, at least in the short term, if that is your main objective. As a result, you will reap all of the health benefits that are associated with carrying fewer pounds – from reduced risk of heart disease to less joint pain. However, all too often, they prioritise cutting calories at the expense of good nutrition, and that can do more harm than good over the long term.

The ManFood plan is different because it does not focus solely on cutting calories. Nevertheless, with a little adaptation, it can still be a highly effective way to lose weight: simply stick to the suggested menus but reduce the size of the portions until you reach your target weight. Then you can start to eat a little more, safe in the knowledge that you are getting all the nutrients you need from a healthy, well-balanced, sustainable diet.

Gaining weight

Almost invariably, weight is discussed in terms of how to lose it. Yet, some people are dangerously underweight and find it almost impossible to gain even a single pound. Needless to say, they don't receive much sympathy, but it can be a serious problem.

If you fall into this category, my best advice is to see a nutritional professional. Your GP may be able to refer you to a dietitian, or you could consult with one privately. You should look for someone who has studied nutrition to degree level for at least three years. (This is important, as some nutritionists' 'qual-ifications' amount to no more than a one-year online course.) They will be able to offer advice on how to manage your weight while meeting all of your nutritional requirements.

USING TECHNOLOGY TO LOSE WEIGHT

You probably own a smartphone and may well have a smart-watch, too. This means that you will be able to download an app with which you can log your calorie intake. Some of the more sophisticated apps also provide a breakdown of the carbs, protein and fat that are contained in any given meal or snack. They are easy to find and use, and the calorie tracking function is usually free.

The first time I used one of these apps, I must admit that I found it irritating to record everything I had eaten or drunk during the week. However, it was worth the effort, because I soon learned precisely how many calories I was consuming. As you might expect, my diet was pretty healthy, but I was surprised by *how much* I was eating. Having the app helped me scale down my portion sizes at main meals and recognise that I was consuming far too many calories in the form of snacks and glasses of red wine.

At first, whenever I identified a portion size that was about the right amount of calories, I took a picture of it so that I could refer to the image in the future. However, after a week or so, I didn't bother with the camera, as more modest portions became second nature. After another week, I didn't even need to use the app too much.

That said, the information it provided in those first couple of weeks has proved invaluable ever since, because it helped me to reframe how much I was eating and gain a greater appreciation of the amount of calories in every meal. It could do the same for you, so it's certainly worth giving it a go.

CHAPTER 6

Energy and stress

Why balancing the two is so important

Energy

I sometimes marvel at how much energy I used to have and how much I got done. I could easily work all day without taking a break, then go straight out, and I would not start to feel tired until much later in the evening. In addition, I would exercise most days, playing energetic games of tennis or going to the gym.

That's all different now that I'm in my mid-fifties. My energy levels aren't what they were, and I know that I have to factor in rest, sleep and recovery after a big event or a night out. However, I take some comfort from the fact that it is entirely normal to have less energy as we age. The mechanism by which the human body makes energy is highly complex and linked to a multitude of factors, many of which start to change as we enter middle age.

Mitochondria reduction

Mitochondria are minuscule structures that are found in nearly every cell in the human body and play a pivotal role in energy production. However, the numbers vary from cell to cell, with muscles typically having the highest concentrations of mito-chondria, whereas inactive fat cells have far fewer.

There's no need to understand the intricacies of the biochem-ical process. You just need to know that mitochondria 'burn' the end products of the food you eat to make a form of energy called adenosine triphosphate (or ATP for short) that can be stored and is then readily available whenever you need it. When energy demands are repeatedly high, then cells adapt to increase the number of mitochondria, enabling them to produce more energy. Conversely, if you are generally inactive, your energy requirements will be low and so cells can respond by decreasing the concentration of mitochondria. Therefore, given that we tend to move less and often become more sedentary as we age, it follows that our cells will start to lose mitochondria, result-ing in less energy. It's a chicken and egg situation, but it can be addressed, at least to some extent, by staying active and engaging in regular sport or exercise.

In addition, the mitochondria become less efficient as we age, which we experience as less energy. This is linked to the fact that all cells have to replicate themselves at regular intervals. In our younger years, the copies are virtually identical to the originals, but over time they become less and less perfect. The theory is that free radicals have ever more opportunities to damage the cells' DNA (their blueprint, if you like) as the years go by, resulting in increasingly flawed copies. Think of this process in terms of taking a photocopy of a photocopy of a photocopy: the image becomes less clear every time.

Reduced blood flow

A slight reduction in blood flow is another natural aspect of the ageing process. This starts to occur in many men around the age of 45. Specifically, the amount of blood that flows in the hepatic portal vein, which serves the gastrointestinal tract, pancreas, gallbladder and spleen, naturally declines over time. Given that this is the blood vessel that carries many of the nutrients that are derived from the food you eat, any reduction in blood flow is likely to have a knock-on effect on energy levels.

Decreasing muscle mass

As I mentioned at the start of Chapter 5, men are naturally endowed with greater muscle mass than women. Although a degree of age-related decline is inevitable and unavoidable, the effects can be mitigated by remaining active. Remember, muscles contain more mitochondria than other cells, and those mito-chondria multiply when energy demands are high. Therefore, it's a good idea to incorporate regular weight-training or strengthen-ing exercises into your weekly routine. This might mean lifting weights in the gym or simply using your own body weight as resistance (for example, by doing push-ups or squats). Your muscles will respond by increasing their mitochondria, which in turn will have a positive effect on your energy levels.

Digestive inefficiency

Everything you chew and swallow passes down the throat and into the stomach, where it is exposed to the powerful effects of hydro-chloric acid, which continues the process of digestion by breaking the bonds that hold the food's chemical compounds together. This involves churning the food to allow the acid to reach every part of it, resulting in a gel-like substance called 'chyme', which then passes from the stomach into the duodenum and the small intestine.

However, hydrochloric acid production declines with age, which can have a knock-on effect on how efficiently you extract certain nutrients from food. The nutrients that seem to be most affected are B12, calcium, iron and beta-carotene. It should be pointed out that the decline in stomach acid, in itself, is unlikely to lead to deficiency in any of these nutrients, but even a small reduction in the amount we are able to absorb may contribute to reduced energy levels.

Stomach acid starts to fall very gradually from around the age of 45, but it is unlikely to cause problems before the age of 65. A digestive enzyme supplement may help (see Chapter 9 for more details), but make sure that you discuss this first with your GP and/or a nutritional professional.

Sleep deprivation

As we saw in Chapter 4, duration and quality of sleep are closely associated with energy levels. First, and most obviously, our energy requirements fall dramatically while we are asleep, so getting insufficient sleep means that we use more energy over longer periods of time. Energy production is finite, so it follows that vigour declines in the sleep-deprived. Furthermore, levels of testosterone and human growth hormone tend to fall as a result of poor and inadequate sleep, which also has a negative impact on energy levels.

Thyroid function

The thyroid gland is located in the lower part of the neck and has several important functions, including producing hormones that tell the human body how much energy to use. If it secretes insufficient amounts of these hormones – a condition known as hypothyroidism in severe cases – symptoms may include a lack of energy, feeling cold, muscle weakness and weight gain.

Although hypothyroidism affects more women than men, it is more likely to occur in both sexes after the age of 50. Therefore, it is sensible to get your GP to check your thyroid regularly from middle age onwards, especially as several of the most common symptoms, including lack of energy, might be dismissed as natural parts of the ageing process. Reduced thyroid function can be treated with medication, but it should be noted that the gland relies on iodine to produce its hormones, so ensuring adequate consumption of that nutrient is a logical first step to decreasing your risk of developing the condition.

As with almost every nutrient, it is preferable to get your iodine from a well-balanced diet, rather than supplements. Most of us need only modest amounts, and it is readily available in seafood, salt-water fish, sea vegetables and some dairy products, especially if the herd's feed has been supplemented with the nutrient (this is often highlighted on the packaging). By contrast, high-strength supplements may result in excess iodine that can exacerbate certain autoimmune conditions that affect the thyroid, such as Hashimoto's thyroiditis.

Energy-boosting nutrients

It could be argued that *all* nutrients have some role to play in the body's production of energy, but a few stand out.

As we saw in Chapter 5, the major food groups – carbs, protein and fat – are metabolised at different rates, which reflects their individual structures and the processes that are required to break them down and extract their fuel. All of this is governed by several factors and practically every nutrient there is, not least a core group of eleven that play a pivotal role in the biochemical conversion of what you eat into substances that can be used in the Krebs cycle. This is the name that is given to the sequence of chemical reactions that takes place in the mitochondria to produce ATP – the packets of energy that are needed by every cell in the body.

It would take an entire book to explain the specific roles of each of these nutrients in this process. Suffice to say here that all eleven are essential to the maintenance of good energy levels, especially later in life. With that in mind, I have compiled a list of the best food sources for each of them. (Once again, I recommend getting these nutrients from your diet, rather than supplements.)

Biotin
- Liver
- Fish
- Egg yolk
- Soya beans
- Hazelnuts
- Almonds
- Swiss chard
- Sweet potato
- Tomato
- Carrots
- Avocado

Folic acid
- Liver
- Pulses (especially lentils, chickpeas and kidney beans)
- Cos lettuce
- Avocado
- Asparagus
- Spinach
- Broccoli

B1 (thiamine)
- Sunflower seeds
- Haricot beans
- Pork
- Barley
- Peas
- Lentils
- Oats
- Wheatgerm

B2 (riboflavin)
- Soya beans
- Spinach
- Yoghurt
- Eggs
- Almonds
- Turkey
- Red meat
- Dark chicken meat
- Quinoa
- Rye

B3 (niacin)

- Poultry
- Fish
- Dairy
- Eggs

- Sweet potato
- Asparagus
- Dates
- Avocado

B5 (pantothenic acid)

- Liver
- Kidney
- Poultry
- Lentils
- Red meat
- Dairy

- Avocado
- Shiitake mushrooms
- Portobello mushrooms
- Tomato paste and purée
- Sunflower seeds
- Sweet potato

B6 (pyridoxine)

- Poultry
- Red meat
- Pulses (especially chickpeas)
- Fish
- Wholegrains
- Brown rice
- Spinach

- Asparagus
- Avocado
- Leeks
- Onions
- Sweet potato
- Bananas
- Cantaloupe melon

B12

Unusually, neither animals nor plants manufacture vitamin B12. Instead, it originates among bacteria, fungi and algae. Yet, it is found in almost all animal tissue as well as several vegetables.

It is also atypical because its method of absorption in the human body is different from those of the other B vitamins. A combination of stomach acid and gastric intrinsic factor (a substance secreted by the stomach's parietal cells) allows B12 to be absorbed further along the digestive tract.

The best food sources are:

- Red meat
- Liver
- Oily fish
- Eggs

- Dairy products (especially yoghurt)
- Fermented foods

Zinc

- Beef
- Lamb
- Sesame seeds
- Game
- Poultry
- Liver
- Eggs
- Seafood

- Seaweed
- Cheese
- Yoghurt
- Nuts
- Oats
- Brown rice
- Pumpkin

Iron

- Liver
- Beef
- Lamb
- Venison
- Chickpeas
- Beans
- Peas

- Chard
- Spinach
- Dried apricots
- Tomato paste and purée
- Curry powder
- Ginger

Copper

- Shellfish
- Offal
- Miso
- Sesame seeds
- Sunflower seeds
- Coconut milk

- Avocado
- Asparagus
- Garlic
- Chestnut mushrooms
- Soya beans
- Oat bran

Stress

You may be wondering why I decided to combine stress and energy in this chapter. Well, they are closely linked, because how you handle stress can have far-reaching effects on general health and particularly energy levels.

Stress is inevitable for all of us at certain times, but the human body is well equipped to deal with it by secreting three powerful hormones – adrenaline, noradrenaline and cortisol – that have a significant impact on many bodily functions (see below). However, this response, which evolved over millions of years, was much more appropriate when our ancestors spent their time hunting for food (and being hunted themselves). Most of us are unlikely to face this sort of imminent danger today, yet exactly the same 'fight or flight' response is still triggered whenever we find ourselves in a stressful meeting, traffic jam, family event or indeed any circumstance that causes acute worry and concern.

Adrenaline and noradrenaline

All forms of stress prompt the adrenal glands to secrete adrenaline and noradrenaline, two hormones that prepare the body to address the situation by prioritising a number of possibly life-saving functions over others that are less urgent:

- Air passages dilate to allow the lungs to take in more oxygen.
- Pupils dilate to improve vision.
- The liver releases stored glucose to meet short-term energy demands.
- The blood thickens to reduce bleeding in the event of injury.

- Increased blood flow to the brain promotes clear thinking.
- Insulin levels fall as the stress hormones make cells less sensitive to its action, so more glucose is available for energy.

As both adrenaline and noradrenaline trigger these responses, for simplicity I will refer to the two hormones simply as 'adrenaline' from now on. They provide a useful surge of energy and focus, which helped our ancestors to avoid falling prey to packs of lions and help us to perform any number of day-to-day tasks. However, part of this process involves the diversion of blood and energy away from 'non-essential' functions, including digestion and the immune system. This may explain why digestive problems and infections – both of which are linked to inflammatory substances in the blood (see Chapter 7) – are particularly common among people who suffer long-term stress.

Cortisol

The other hormone that is secreted at times of stress is cortisol, albeit with less urgency than adrenaline. It is naturally produced every morning, with levels gradually decreasing as the day progresses, although stress can cause spikes at any time, and these can have negative effects over the long term.

Most cells in the body have cortisol receptors, so it has wider effects than adrenaline, which is more targeted in its action. It helps to stabilise blood glucose levels, reduces inflammation, is involved in regulating metabolism and affects sodium and potassium levels, so it has the potential to increase blood pressure.

However, excessive production of cortisol over a prolonged period of time (by which I mean several years) can lead to a condition called Cushing's syndrome. Symptoms include loss of bone density, dangerously high blood pressure, fatigue, muscle weakness and weight gain, especially around the face and abdomen. By contrast, too little cortisol can lead to Addison's disease, which is also typified by muscle weakness and fatigue as well as dizziness and weight loss. Both of these conditions require medical attention and probably consultation with an endocrinologist.

In times of extreme and/or prolonged stress, cortisol and adrenaline can be released at inappropriate times, such as in the early hours of the morning, leading to sudden wakening with a racing mind and an elevated heart rate. It might be more than an hour before these effects subside and sleep is possible again, which obviously causes tiredness the following day and increases the likelihood of gravitating towards foods with a high fat and sugar content (see Chapter 4).

The long-term effects of stress

It is quite possible that stress worked well for you in your youth. After all, the stress hormones allow you to work and function with greater focus and energy. In fact, many young people *like* to feel stressed and use adrenaline to their advantage.

However, prolonged stress over the course of many years, which results in excessive levels of cortisol and adrenaline in the bloodstream, is widely associated with some serious health problems, including heart disease and prostate issues. In all likelihood, such conditions are either caused or at least exacerbated by the inflammatory effects of these stress hormones. The next chapter covers inflammation in much more detail, but for now we need to concentrate on how to keep stress under control, as this will help to reduce inflammation throughout the body.

Stress relief through diet and supplementation

If you were to go online and search for 'nutrients and stress', you would be presented with a list of vitamins and minerals that are said to ameliorate stress. For instance, vitamins B5 and C, curcumin, the minerals zinc and magnesium and omega 3 fats are frequently cited as effective stress-busters.

However, when you dig deeper into the research, you find that the studies into these nutrients' efficacy are usually based on supplementation rather than natural food sources. (It is standard practice in some medical research to prescribe large doses of particular nutrients when attempting to establish some sort of correlation between them and certain conditions.) For example, several studies have reported retardation of cortisol production among athletes who are given high doses of vitamin C in supplement form. Similarly, another trial found that the stress response in rats that were supplemented with 200mg of vitamin C a day declined significantly. These results may seem promising, but the amount of vitamin C the rats were given was equivalent to several grams in human terms. It would be impossible to consume such large quantities without supplementation, regardless of how many vitamin C-rich foods you ate.

That said, it seems that the adrenal glands secrete vitamin C along with cortisol, so it is logical to replenish your reserves of this important vitamin, especially at times of stress. Therefore, this is one of the few occasions when there is a valid argument for medium or even high-dose supplementation, given the findings of the aforementioned reports. The same is true for zinc: several studies suggest that it can slow cortisol production and reduce the hormone's harmful effects, but only when taken in large quantities in supplement form which is definitely not advisable.

Magnesium is rather different, as it can dampen the influence of the stress hormones, rather than slow their production and release.

This is because, as we saw in Chapter 4, it is a key component in GABA – the neurotransmitter that sends messages throughout the nervous system and into the brain. I often recommend a 100mg or 200mg supplement last thing at night for clients who are struggling to sleep due to chronic stress. In addition, this sort of dose will ease bowel movements, which can be useful as constipation is another common symptom of long-term stress. It is also involved in the production of the 'feelgood hormones' dopamine and serotonin, both of which can help to alleviate stress. See page 122 for a list of the foods that are rich in magnesium.

Another nutrient that plays an important role in GABA production is the amino acid theanine, which is found almost exclusively in tea. The general rule of thumb is the stronger the tea, the more theanine it will contain, be it black, green, white or red (although black contains more than the others). On the other hand, the longer you leave your tea to brew, the more caffeine you will drink, which could increase your stress (see below). I think the best compromise is to enjoy moderate-strength tea, or switch to decaffeinated as the level of theanine is unaffected by the decaffeination process.

Caffeine

Just as stress triggers the release of adrenaline, so does caffeine. Of course, this can be useful, as it provides a rapid, short-term surge of energy. Yet it also encourages the production of cortisol, which may magnify feelings of stress and increase the risk of associated health problems over the long term. In addition, remember that the brain's adenosine receptors become increasingly desensitised over time, reducing the stimulant effect of the caffeine and the hormones, but a cup of coffee will continue to encourage the same amount of cortisol production.

Glucose levels

In the last chapter, we saw that eating 'little and often' is one of the best ways to maintain equilibrium in your level of blood glucose. This could play an important role in stress management because one of the principal functions of adrenaline and cortisol is to step in and raise glucose if the body's demands for fuel are not being met. Therefore, eating modest amounts throughout the day might eliminate at least one of the main reasons why the stress hormones are released.

Alcohol

Most of us are well aware of the potential pleasures of alcohol, but did you know that it can also trigger the release of adrenaline and cortisol? Indeed, it has been suggested that the initial sensation of well-being you may experience when drinking is connected to the stimulating effects of these stress hormones. However, the sensation is dulled through frequent and especially excessive exposure to alcohol. Consequently, light and/or occasional drinkers are likely to experience it far more readily than those who drink heavily and often.

Alcohol may also be detrimental to sleep quality (see Chapter 4), which can be especially problematic at times of stress.

Reducing stress

A few years ago, during an especially stressful period in my life, I decided to cut out all caffeine and alcohol, as I felt that both were magnifying my anxiety. I am confident that the sacrifice was worthwhile (although there's no way to prove it), and you may wish to try a similar experiment if you are feeling under stress. On the other hand, other approaches might be just as effective.

For example, one study reported a 7 per cent reduction in cortisol levels among a group of men who started to practise regular meditation. Moreover, that figure rose to 22 per cent among a more experienced group. Finding the time for meditation might seem impossible, but the benefits can be profound, so it is certainly worth trying. For instance, it can help you feel brighter, improve your focus and concentration, and even promote longer and better sleep. There is no shortage of groups, private teachers, apps and classes, so it should be easy to find one that suits your particular preferences and requirements.

Alternatively, or in addition, you could try gardening, walking, socialising, board games, cooking, yoga, jigsaw puzzles or fishing. In fact, anything that provides a few minutes or hours of distraction from the stresses of everyday life can be very beneficial.

And, of course, follow the ManFood plan to ensure you eat a healthy diet, because life is stressful enough without worrying about whether you are getting all the nutrients you need.

CHAPTER 7

Inflammation

An important yet overlooked issue

You don't hear much about it, but inflammation is a significant factor in a wide variety of serious health complaints, including heart disease, deteriorating cognitive function, type 2 diabetes, asthma, prostate issues, low energy, poor stress response and erectile dysfunction. Moreover, even if you don't suffer from any of these conditions, it probably manifests itself in your daily life in one way or another, be it in the form of a headache, arthritis, toothache, blocked sinuses or sore throat. Yet, we rarely associate these issues with inflammation, so we tend to underestimate the damage it is causing. In addition, there is evidence that all of the problems associated with inflammation – be they serious or minor – tend to increase as we get older, so it is an especially important subject for anyone over the age of 45.

It can be difficult to understand how inflammation operates inside the body, so an all too familiar example may help. Say you accidentally bang your finger with a hammer. You will expect it to turn red, throb and swell – three effects that may last a few hours or even a day or two before the swelling subsides and the colour returns largely to normal, aside from a residual bruise. All of this is linked to inflammation. At the precise moment when the weight of the hammer hits your thumb, your immune system responds by releasing a variety of chemical compounds, collectively known as 'mediators of inflammation'. These include histamine, nitric oxide and a group of fatty substances called prostaglandins (hormones that help the blood to clot and seal off the injured area), along with white blood cells, which absorb and eliminate the damaged cells. Meanwhile, cells in the vicinity of the damaged thumb produce molecules called cytokines. These aid communication and interact with the immune cells to regulate their response. Some of them also stimulate the production of more mediators of inflammation, while others halt this process as soon as the situation is under control.

In addition to springing into life when there is an injury, the immune system responds to invasion by foreign bodies, such as viruses or bacteria. However, in contrast to their response to a sudden injury, such as a hammer blow to the thumb, any immune cells that identify an invader will try to fight it themselves before calling for back-up. This is why a toothache often starts with a slight tingle or warm sensation. It's only later, when the back-up arrives and the whole area becomes more inflamed, that the pain ramps up. In the ensuing battle, infected cells and invaders alike will be killed and injured – a conflict that may well be visible in the form of pus. However, once victory over the invader has been secured, the whole area will be cleared and normal service can resume.

When the stimulus for immune response is chronic (that is, it persists for a prolonged period of time), including long-term injuries and autoimmune conditions, the process is slightly different. This is because the various mediators of inflammation remain ever present, continuing to do their jobs amid the damaged cells and tissue, while white blood cells attempt to resolve the problem and clear away the detritus.

Now, imagine inflammation inside the body, triggered by

some internal damage or threat, such as oxidation or a toxin. In Chapter 1, we saw that cholesterol tends to stick to damaged and inflamed areas of the intima (the lining of the blood vessels). Therefore, in this classic example of chronic inflammation, the body's ongoing attempts to contain and repair physical damage leads to hardening and less flexibility. Hence, inflammation is an important factor in atherosclerosis.

However, chronic inflammation isn't always associated with a specific part of the body, such as the intima. Sometimes, it can affect the whole body. For example, obese people obviously have far more fat cells than those who are a healthy weight. Like all other cells in the human body, fat cells produce various molecules that influence the production of glucose, how dietary fats are processed and the way in which energy is used. Therefore, if the number of fat cells in the abdomen reaches unusually high levels, this can result in the overproduction of cytokines and mediators of inflammation. In turn, the liver will respond by producing more of a substance called C-reactive protein (CRP), which can be measured via a blood test to establish the level of inflammation.

Inflammatory cytokines and associated substances are potential factors in benign prostate enlargement, impaired cognitive function, depression, some forms of cancer, bone loss and possibly even weight gain. Bear in mind that the progression of any disease that is linked to inflammation tends to be gradual but relentless, with the damage increasing over time. Men and women are equally affected by inflammation, but there is some evidence that low testosterone later in life may be linked to higher levels of a number of inflammatory agents.

Given the widespread damage that this silent threat can cause, it is logical to do whatever you can to reduce inflammation, starting with your diet.

Nutrition and inflammation

Avoid sugar and simple carbs

As I have just mentioned, obesity can be a major contributor to inflammation, so it is important to keep your weight under control. See Chapter 5 for detailed advice on how to achieve this.

In the same chapter, we learned that simple carbs, such as white pasta, bread, cakes, confectionery and many cereals, are broken down relatively easily. By contrast, complex carbs' journey from food to glucose is much slower, because the digestive system has to separate their sugars from fibre. In addition, we learned that eating complex carbs with protein and a little fat results in a slow and steady supply of glucose. By contrast, eating simple carbs and sugar on their own, in isolation from protein and fibre, causes rapid spikes in blood glucose levels, and consequently elevated levels of insulin. This hormone drives glucose into the cells, where it is used as fuel to make energy, and shunts away any excess for conversion into fat, which is then stored in the body. However, inflammation can reduce cells' sensitivity to insulin, a condition that is known as 'insulin resistance'. This can have a detrimental effect on energy levels and result in the conversion of even more glucose into fat, which in turn exacerbates inflammation. It's a vicious circle.

Therefore, you should aim for a diet that favours fibre-rich, complex carbs and protein over simple carbs as this will help you to regulate glucose production and avoid insulin resistance. Meanwhile, reducing inflammation in general can enhance insulin sensitivity.

METABOLIC SYNDROME

'Metabolic syndrome' (or 'Syndrome X') is an umbrella term for five conditions that were first identified and linked some ninety years ago, although the term itself was not coined until the 1980s. The five conditions are:

- high blood pressure;
- obesity;
- raised triglycerides;
- low HDL cholesterol; and
- insulin resistance.

If you have any three of these, you may be diagnosed with metabolic syndrome, and categorised as having an increased risk of heart disease, stroke and type 2 diabetes.

Inflammation is a factor in developing the syndrome, as is a low level of testosterone, which becomes more likely as we age.

Dietary fats

In Chapter 3, we looked at the important role played by some dietary fats in maintaining cognitive function, but there is also a direct link between the fats you eat and inflammation.

Saturated fats

First and foremost, saturated fats seem to encourage the production of mediators of inflammation. These fats are found in dairy products, such as butter, cream, full-fat milk and ghee, fatty cuts of meat, processed meats, including salami and sausages, and lard. We do need *some* saturated fat in our diet, which is why these foods appear from time to time in the ManFood plan. However, the standard Western diet provides far too much.

Trans fats

Trans fats can interfere with the ways in which cells communicate with each other, which can result in significant overproduction of cytokines and other inflammatory substances. Therefore, they are best avoided.

Omega 3 and 6

While omega 3 fats are known to discourage inflammation, omega 6 fats have the opposite effect by dampening their close cousins' anti-inflammatory impact. This is unfortunate because the standard Western diet contains large amounts of omega 6 and insufficient omega 3. For example, omega 6 is found in poultry, eggs, nuts, seeds, vegetable oils, pumpkin and sesame seeds and their oils, but also in biscuits, crackers and sweets if they are made with vegetable oil (which many are). By contrast, the best sources of omega 3 are oily fish, such as mackerel and herring, which have largely fallen out of favour.

This is not to say that you should try to avoid omega 6 altogether, because it has many beneficial properties. For instance, nuts are a key food in managing cholesterol, yet many contain omega 6 fats. However, it is certainly advisable to steer clear of vegetable oils, biscuits, sweets and other processed foods, which is why they are not included in the ManFood plan. On the other hand, the plan actively encourages the consumption of more omega 3 on account of its numerous health benefits, including its anti-inflammatory effects.

Vitamin C

There is mounting evidence that even relatively low doses of vitamin C can counteract the overproduction of mediators of inflammation and CRP. For instance, several studies have found that as little as 70mg a day has some anti-inflammatory effect. You will get more than 80mg from one medium-sized orange, 60mg from a single green pepper, 30mg from one spear of broccoli, 64mg from a kiwi fruit and 7mg from a single strawberry. Therefore, it's easy to consume 70mg from diet alone; supplements are unnecessary in this instance. Bear in mind, though, that vitamin C cannot be stored in the body, so you will need to replenish your supply each day.

Vitamin E

Vitamin E also seems to dampen the production of mediators of inflammation. However, it is not quite as simple as that because there are eight different forms of this vitamin, each of which has a slightly different effect. Four of these are known as tocopherols (alpha, beta, gamma and delta), while the other four are termed tocotrienols (again, alpha, beta, gamma and delta). It is alpha- and gamma-tocopherol that affect inflammation, slowing the production of cytokines and mediators of inflammation, including prostaglandins, respectively.

Nevertheless, I do not recommend supplementing vitamin E, because doing so can thin the blood, which in turn may increase the risk of haemorrhagic stroke by as much as 22 per cent. Therefore, you should aim to meet all of your vitamin E needs through diet alone. The following foods are good sources:

- Wheatgerm
- Sunflower seeds
- Almonds
- Salmon

- Avocado
- Trout
- Pumpkin seeds
- Brazil nuts
- Mango
- Kiwi fruit
- Red pepper
- Butternut squash
- Broccoli
- Asparagus
- Olive oil

Polyphenols

'Polyphenols' is an umbrella term for some 8000 plant chemical compounds that have some sort of antioxidant effect. Sub-groups include flavonoids, phenolic acid, isoflavones and lignans. Collectively, they have a multitude of benefits, including significant anti-inflammatory potential, given that oxidation is a major cause of inflammation.

A number of high-quality studies have isolated specific polyphenols and found that they inhibit the production of substances that are known to cause inflammation. However, it should be pointed out that all fruits and vegetables – as well as foodstuffs in which they are the primary ingredients, such as red wine, tea, cocoa and coffee – contain these beneficial chemicals in one form or another, so inflammatory markers such as CRP tend to be reduced *whenever* they are consumed in reasonable quantities on a regular basis. That said, it is worth discussing one particularly good source of polyphenols, not least because it has attracted a great deal of attention over recent years.

You are probably already familiar with turmeric, the bright yellow spice that is often a key ingredient of Indian dishes. This has gained huge popularity among the so-called 'wellness brigade', which includes health bloggers and other enthusiastic users of social media. In part, this is due to the fact that it contains turmerin, turmerone, elemene, furanodiene, curdione, bisacurone and germacrone – all of which are formidable polyphenols in their own right. However, the one that is most relevant in the context of inflammation is curcumin.

Many studies suggest that large doses of this polyphenol can reduce inflammation by inhibiting the activity of cells that are involved in the inflammatory process. Unfortunately, though, it comprises just 5 per cent of the total weight of the spice, so a pinch or two of turmeric in the occasional curry is unlikely to alleviate any of the problems associated with inflammation. In addition, curcumin is poorly absorbed by the body if turmeric is eaten in isolation (although the addition of black pepper can help with this).

All of this means that it is very difficult to get the requisite large quantities of curcumin from food alone, unless you want everything you eat to taste of turmeric. Therefore, it seems that the only practical way to reap any benefit from its much-touted anti-inflammatory properties is to take it in supplement form. However, as ever, I would strongly urge you to consult a qualified nutritionist and your GP beforehand, as they will be able to provide information and advice on all of the potential benefits and drawbacks.

Prebiotics and probiotics

It could be argued that what we know about gut microbiome and its influence on the workings of the human body is still in its infancy (see Chapter 10 for more details). However, in the context of inflammation, there is increasing evidence that it plays an important role in regulating the production of inflammatory cytokines.

Prebiotic foods – such as onions, garlic, Jerusalem artichoke, leeks, asparagus, bananas, oats, apples and cocoa – contain indigestible fibre that ferments as it travels along the digestive tract. By the time it reaches the intestines, this fermented fibre provides sustenance for the beneficial bacteria – also known as probiotics – that live in the gut and therefore helps to maintain optimum gut health. All of these foods also contain a variety of polyphenols, so they are doubly beneficial. A word of warning, however: they can cause bloating and discomfort, especially when consumed in large quantities. For instance, I once deeply regretted having a second (small) bowl of Jerusalem artichoke soup.

The term probiotics is also used to describe both the microorganisms that are found in fermented foods, such as miso and sauerkraut (see Chapter 10 for further details), and certain supplement products, such as yoghurt drinks, that are said to improve gut health (see Chapters 10 and 16 for further details).

CHAPTER 8

Testosterone

A crucial and often overlooked hormone

These days, testosterone, the male sex hormone, tends to be viewed in a rather negative light. For instance, when boys and young men run amok, they are often accused of 'testosterone-fuelled behaviour', as if the hormone's pernicious influence has the power to turn good men bad. This is just one of many ways in which 'testosterone' is used as shorthand for a particularly aggressive form of youthful masculinity. To some extent, the association is justified, because levels of testosterone start to decline naturally from the age of 30 onwards, and thereafter many men do indeed become more placid than they once were.

In addition, though, this hormone plays a crucial role in a wide variety of mental and physical functions, so the age-related downturn in production impacts far more than merely our ability to remain calm. For example:

- Sperm production relies on several hormones, including testosterone, which encourages the cells to mature.
- Male sex hormones, primarily testosterone, help to maintain healthy bone density, so lower levels are linked to an increased risk of fractures in older men.
- Testosterone enhances libido, desire and erections.

- It is also linked to insulin sensitivity and glucose control, so reduced levels can result in larger fat deposits, especially in the abdomen and thighs. (Incidentally, the relationship works both ways, so reducing obesity can help to raise levels of testosterone.)
- Muscle size and strength are both affected by testosterone, probably because it is involved in the metabolism of dietary protein.
- Testosterone increases both the activity and effectiveness of erythropoietin (EPO), a hormone produced by the kidneys that promotes red blood cell production in bone marrow.
- Assertiveness and self-confidence – which should not be confused with aggression or machismo – are both linked to the level of testosterone.
- It is also closely associated with energy, personal ambition and positivity, and may play a role in maintaining cognitive function.

Testosterone through the ages

Testosterone is present in the womb, where it helps to shape the male characteristics of the foetus. Toddlers and young boys have relatively low levels, but these start to increase around the age of 10. They rise gradually for a year or two, but then gather pace, triggering a host of momentous bodily changes, such as maturation of the genitalia and hair growth under the armpits and in the pubic region, as well as the notorious behavioural changes. Thereafter, there are usually two more steep increases around the ages of 16 and 18. Levels then remain steady until the age of 30, whereupon they start falling at a rate of about 1 per cent per year.

You can have a blood test to measure your level of testosterone, but the results can be misleading due to the presence of a substance called sex-hormone binding globulin (SHBG), which, as the name suggests, binds itself to both male and female hormones. This can have a dramatic impact on testosterone's ability to perform its numerous tasks, so, even if the test reports a healthy quantity of the hormone, it may not be functioning correctly. Therefore, should you choose to have a testosterone test, you should also ask the doctor to measure your level of SHBG and, even more importantly, your level of free (unbound) testosterone.

The testosterone debate

Although the decline in testosterone is a natural part of the ageing process, there are ongoing attempts to counteract low levels through the development of testosterone-boosting medication. Of course, this is entirely understandable, given the crucial role that the hormone plays in so many important bodily functions. After all, who wouldn't want to be lean rather than have middle-aged spread or prefer youthful vigour to perpetual fatigue? Male testosterone deficiency (TD) is now a recognised medical condition that is said to affect some 9 per cent of all middle-aged men (and some 24 per cent of those with type 2 diabetes), so it's hardly surprising that the big pharmaceutical companies are all competing with one another to provide the most effective treatment.

In addition, though, while TD is undeniably a serious condition that should be addressed, simply restoring testosterone to the levels that we all 'enjoyed' as teenagers is increasingly presented as a panacea for a whole host of familiar health – and especially sexual – issues. Consequently, ever more men are asking if something can be done about their 'low T', and it is possible that more doctors are giving serious consideration to the idea of prescribing 'testosterone replacement therapy', even for men whose levels are entirely consistent with their age. Nevertheless, at present, most men do not qualify for medical intervention on the NHS without first receiving a diagnosis of clinical deficiency.

You might find this information disappointing, but should bear in mind that more testosterone may not be the answer anyway. Common problems such as fatigue, weight gain, low mood and lack of drive could be due to a malfunctioning thyroid, depression, excess weight or too much alcohol, among many other causes, rather than 'low T'. None of these potential causes should be discounted, and they should all be factored in and addressed prior to putting the blame on testosterone.

Testosterone replacement therapy

Testosterone replacement therapy comes in three forms: injection, oral medication and a gel that is rubbed on the skin. All three are effective, but they are not without their risks. For example, even though testosterone is required to maintain fertility, replacement therapy can lead to *infertility*, because the levels of other hormones that are involved in sperm production tend to fall in response.

It can also affect the prostate gland, which is why most doctors insist on a digital rectal examination and possibly a PSA test before prescribing the therapy. This allows them to establish a base level against which any changes to the prostate may be assessed. In addition, you might develop acne and/or experience some swelling of your breast tissue. While unwelcome, these symptoms are generally harmless and diminish over time, although you should keep your doctor apprised of them.

There was a long-held belief that testosterone replacement

therapy could increase the risk of cardiovascular disease, but this has been largely disproved through meta-analysis of a large number of previous scientific studies. Once again, though, your doctor will be able to offer guidance on the risk in relation to your individual health status and circumstances.

You may have noticed that I have mentioned discussing testosterone replacement therapy with your GP throughout this section. This is very important, because there is a great deal of misinformation out there, especially online, and you should never even consider embarking on this sort of treatment without first seeking professional medical advice. Needless to say, you should also never buy testosterone online. First, you have no way of knowing that what you are buying is even testosterone. Second, the prescribed dosage may be dangerously high, especially if you are suffering from other (possibly undiagnosed) conditions. Third, and most importantly, testosterone is a controlled substance that is regulated by the government, so you could be breaking the law.

Testosterone and nutrition

If you were to go online and search for various nutrients that boost testosterone, you would probably come across countless websites devoted to weightlifting and fitness training. This is because the hormone is frequently viewed as an easy route to building extra muscle and enhancing the results that you would get from exercise alone.

However, the nutritional advice on these websites typically recommends supplements, rather than food, primarily extracts of herbs such as fenugreek and a member of the caltrop family with the scientific name *Tribulus terrestis*. The latter is usually discussed in glowing terms, and various studies tend to be cited to confirm its efficacy in boosting testosterone. Yet, a closer look reveals that these studies are far from scientific, so their findings don't count for much. Indeed, my inner sceptic suspects that all of these products and the accompanying 'evidence' are designed to boost sales, rather than testosterone.

Other trials have suggested that three familiar nutrients – magnesium, vitamin D and zinc – might help to increase levels. Once again, though, the nutrients tend to be delivered in high-dosage supplement form. For example, one frequently cited study gave a group of ten healthy volunteers supplemental zinc at a level of 3mg per kilo of body weight and reported increased testosterone levels in all of the participants. On this basis, given that I weigh around 80 kilos, I would need to take a supplement of 240mg of zinc each day. Yet, the recommended upper limit for zinc intake is just 40mg per day from all sources (food as well as supplements), so supplementing *six times* that amount for any period of time seems positively foolhardy. Indeed, there is a wealth of evidence to suggest that anything in excess of 100mg of zinc per day may cause nausea, diarrhoea, vomiting, an unpleasant metallic taste in the mouth and kidney damage, while also doubling the risk of prostate cancer.

The evidence for the efficacy of vitamin D supplementation in terms of boosting testosterone is also mixed. Nevertheless, given that it is safe (as long as you abide by the recommended daily amount) and has a number of proven health benefits, it is certainly worth trying, especially later in life.

Another widely recommended supplement in relation to testosterone is dehydroepiandrosterone, better known as DHEA. Produced naturally by the adrenal glands, although it performs certain functions in its own right, it is also a precursor to more powerful male and female sex hormones, including testosterone. However, DHEA production starts to decline from the mid-twenties onwards, which may lead to deficiency. In such cases, supplementation is the only answer, as there are no food sources of DHEA.

However, while raising levels of DHEA through supplementation is relatively straightforward, there are no guarantees that the body will then convert it into testosterone. For example, although one meta-analysis reported that supplementation had a 'small but significant' effect on body composition among elderly men, it found no evidence of improvement in sexual function. In addition, while DHEA is sold over the counter as a dietary supplement in the United States, it is only available on prescription in the UK and many other countries. Therefore, you should consult with your GP if you are thinking of placing an order online, as they will offer a much more balanced view than the websites that sell DHEA supplements.

While we're looking at pills and capsules, there is some evidence that statins can have a detrimental effect on testosterone levels, although the exact mechanism by which they do this is yet to be identified. As we saw in Chapter 1, statins are now widely prescribed to reduce cholesterol, especially from middle age onwards. Once again, if you are concerned, you should discuss this with your GP.

Finally, many studies suggest that excessive alcohol consumption over a prolonged period of time can reduce levels of testosterone. So, this is yet another good reason to moderate your intake.

The effects of sleep and weight loss on testosterone

There is no doubt that maintaining a healthy weight has a beneficial effect on testosterone levels. We know that testosterone is closely associated with another hormone, insulin, and glucose management, so being overweight has an unwelcome effect on all three. Therefore, losing weight can restore testosterone to normal, healthy levels. See Chapter 5 for more information on weight, insulin and glucose management.

Similarly, it seems that sleep deprivation may lower testosterone, while longer and better-quality sleep can help to restore levels.

CHAPTER 9

Your bones

Don't take them for granted

Osteoporosis is a condition in which bones lose tissue, which in turn makes them more brittle and susceptible to fracturing. This is widely but erroneously viewed as a 'women's issue', primarily because levels of oestrogen – the collective term for a group of hormones that not only regulate the female reproductive system but also provide some protection against osteoporosis – decline dramatically during the menopause. As a result, women are indeed more prone to the condition during middle age.

However, men are not immune to osteoporosis. Our bone density starts to deteriorate around the age of 35, and by 65 or 70, on average, it is little better than women's. Therefore, it's important for everyone – men as well as women – to ensure that their diet contains sufficient quantities of several key nutrients that keep bones healthy.

THE STRUCTURE OF BONES

You might think of a bone as hard and solid, but the centre is filled with marrow and nerve cells that are held in a fibrous substance called collagen. This means that bones are strong, light and flexible living structures. In addition, they store 99 per cent of the body's calcium and 85 per cent of its phosphorous.

Cells called osteoblasts manufacture all of the bones in the human body out of a substance called hydroxylapatite, a form of calcium. Meanwhile, cells called osteoclasts break down existing bones to release their stored calcium in a process known as demineralising. Therefore, osteoblasts and osteoclasts are engaged in a constant remodelling of the body's skeleton.

Osteoporosis in men

Statistically, women are at greater risk of developing osteoporosis, but this is mostly explained by the fact that it is age-related: the longer you live, the more likely you are to suffer from the condition. And, on average, women in the UK live four years longer than men (eighty-three as opposed to seventy-nine years).

Nevertheless, according to an International Osteoporosis Foundation report published in 2014, the condition affects one in five men as well as one in three women. Furthermore, the report states that men are more likely than women to die following a hip fracture (one of the more common osteoporosis-related injuries) and points out that 'the lifetime risk of experiencing an osteoporotic fracture in men over the age of 50 is up to 27 per cent higher than the lifetime risk of developing prostate cancer'.

In addition, those over 70 are 50 per cent more likely to suffer a fracture than younger men. Finally, it concludes that men's risk of developing osteoporosis is likely to increase in the future.

Post-menopausal women are routinely tested for osteoporosis, whereas men are not, unless they suffer a fracture, back pain or loss of height. Therefore, it may be prudent to request a check-up, especially as the condition itself is painless and therefore undetectable without testing, if only to establish a baseline against which any changes may be measured.

The most common causes of osteoporosis in men

There are many possible reasons why your bones may lose density, above and beyond the inevitable decline due to ageing.

There are two types of osteoporosis: primary and secondary. Primary osteoporosis refers to age-related loss of bone density, usually in men over 70, as well as inexplicable bone loss in younger men. Meanwhile, the more common secondary osteoporosis is linked to an existing medical condition, medication or some other factor, such as the four potential causes that are discussed below.

Hypogonadism

As testosterone levels fall naturally with age, so does bone density, so it might seem logical that supplementing testosterone would encourage osteoblasts to strengthen the body's bones. However, testosterone replacement therapy has mixed results in this respect, with some studies demonstrating only a moderate improvement in bone density in some bones and others no effect whatsoever.

As far as we can tell, the success of testosterone replacement therapy in promoting bone density depends on several factors, including length of time that testosterone levels have been low, age, lifestyle and the presence of other medications. Your GP should take all of these factors into account when assessing if there is any connection between your level of testosterone and osteoporosis, and therefore whether you would benefit from the therapy.

Glucocorticoids

Steroid medications known as glucocorticoids are widely used to manage inflammatory conditions such as asthma, rheumatoid arthritis and other autoimmune complaints. However, they can have several serious side-effects, including reducing the amount of calcium that the body can absorb from the intestines. If this happens and you become calcium deficient, your osteoclasts are left with no option but to demineralise your bones, given that 99 per cent of your reserves of this mineral are stored there. This usually occurs within the first six months of starting gluco-corticoid treatment.

The link between glucocorticoids and osteoporosis is so well established that many doctors now prescribe an additional medication (such as risedronic acid in a once-a-week pill) to offset the risk of bone damage when treating autoimmune conditions. Simply increasing your intake of calcium and supplementing vitamin D may help, too, but these may be inadequate in themselves. Therefore, you should always discuss what is required with your GP.

Alcohol

While there is a wealth of information regarding the relationship between certain medications and bone density, the precise link between alcohol and bone damage is less clear-cut. Nevertheless, there does seem to be a correlation. This may be due to the fact that alcohol has the potential to hinder the absorption of certain minerals during digestion. In addition, excessive consumption of alcohol can harm liver function and therefore interfere with the conversion of vitamin D into its active form.

Logic dictates that either or both of these may be factors in loss of bone density, although as yet we cannot be sure which of them has the greater influence. Nevertheless, it does seem that, while light drinking can help to increase bone density, heavy drinking has the opposite effect. In this case, light drinking is defined as no more than two units a day (i.e. one 175ml glass of wine or a generous shot of spirit).

Incidentally, statistics suggest that men's risk of suffering a fracture after consuming too much alcohol is slightly greater than women's. Maybe women are simply better at keeping their balance, but it is certainly feasible that men in that state have brittle bones as a result of years of heavy drinking.

Smoking

I smoked long into my twenties, but finally gave up when the health risks became impossible to ignore. Nevertheless, while I haven't smoked for thirty years, my risk of developing osteoporosis is still significantly higher than it would have been if I'd never started (although not nearly as high as that of someone who is *still* smoking).

There is no doubt that smoking is closely associated with the loss of bone density, although we are not sure why. It may be that nicotine is detrimental to mineral absorption. On the other hand, smokers also tend to take less exercise, drink more alcohol and are more likely to be underweight than non-smokers, all of which are significant risk factors for osteoporosis in themselves.

Nutrients that can help to maintain bone density

Calcium

Most people are well aware that calcium is essential for the maintenance of healthy bones. Indeed, it is so important that the body has a system that is specifically designed to maintain optimum levels. The parathyroid glands sit just behind the thyroid gland at the base of neck, but they are otherwise unrelated and have separate functions. These glands constantly monitor calcium levels in the blood and secrete parathyroid hormone (PTH) if they detect any fall. This hormone travels to the bones, where it stimulates the release of stored calcium until levels return to normal. Therefore, whenever the body's calcium requirements are not met through the diet, the bones are mined for their reserves, which is obviously something that you should try to avoid.

Unfortunately, levels of stomach acid may start to decline from about the age of 55 onwards (see below), which can make it increasingly difficult to absorb a range of minerals, including calcium. Consequently, if you are over 55, you should aim to consume at least 1200mg of calcium each day (20 per cent more than you need earlier in life). A supplement may help you achieve this (see Chapter 16), although, as ever, the better option is to meet all of your requirements through the food you eat, which in this case is perfectly feasible. In addition, many of the calcium-rich foods listed in the box below are good sources of vitamin D, so they are doubly beneficial.

The best dietary sources of calcium

The table below gives the amount of calcium per standard portion size.

Food	Portion size	Amount of calcium
Sardines	100g	460mg
Pilchards	Small tin	250mg
Tofu	100g	510mg
Almonds	15g	40mg
Spinach	80g	130mg
Spring greens	80g	60mg
Watercress	50g	85mg
Milk	Medium glass	250mg
Yoghurt	100g	120mg
Cheddar cheese	30g	210mg
Baked beans	Small can	80mg
Kidney beans	100g	70mg

Three common dietary substances can hinder the absorption of calcium: tannins, which are found in tea and coffee; phytates, which are found in bran, beans and some nuts and seeds; and oxalates, which are found in spinach, almonds, peanuts and some soft fruits. However, their impact is quite modest, and they are often found alongside some highly beneficial nutrients (including calcium itself), so it is not necessary to exclude any of these foodstuffs. Just be aware of the effect they can have and maybe increase your intake of calcium from other sources accordingly.

Alternatively, it might be worth trying probiotics, specifically some strains of *Lactobacillus* and *Bifidobacterium*, as there is some evidence that these can increase calcium absorption and therefore offset any reduction caused by phytates and oxalates (see Chapter 10 for more details). By contrast, excess salt intake can promote calcium *excretion*, which is just one of the many reasons why you should exercise discretion when adding it to food (others include well-established links to cardiovascular disease and high blood pressure).

Meanwhile, high-protein diets can increase the body's demand for calcium. You may have read that the phosphoric acid in carbonated drinks can have a negative impact on calcium levels, which is true, to a certain extent. But there is far more phosphoric acid in protein-rich foods such as chicken than there is in a can of cola. As long as you don't go overboard on either, and make sure you hit your 1200mg target each day, your calcium levels should be fine.

Vitamin D

In Chapter 2, we looked at vitamin D's role in preventing prostate inflammation, but it is just as important in maintaining bone density, because it is directly involved in the process of calcium absorption in the intestines.

An inactive form of Vitamin D is made in the skin in response to sunlight. This is then activated by PTH in the kidneys. Therefore, you should try to get about twenty minutes of direct sunlight each day, without wearing sunblock. (This sort of modest exposure without protection is considered perfectly safe in the UK, given the relative weakness of the sun.) Ideally, you would bare your chest, or at least your shoulders, to maximise your exposure to the sun's UV rays, although obviously this is not always practical, especially in the depths of winter. This is one of the reasons why I recommend supplementation of vitamin D, particularly in the winter months. See Chapter 16 for further details.

Vitamin D is also found naturally in some foods, most notably oily fish, soya products and shiitake mushrooms, while other foodstuffs, including some cereals and juices, are fortified with it. By contrast, a very high-protein diet can lead to higher levels of phosphorous, which in turn can interfere with vitamin D synthesis. Of course, I took this into account when compiling the menus and food advice for the ManFood plan.

Magnesium

Low levels of magnesium seem to have an impact on both the production and activity of PTH, which in turn discourages the body's osteoblasts from producing fresh bone, and possibly even encourages osteoclasts to demineralise existing bone.

Magnesium is a key constituent of bone, along with calcium, so we need around 375mg each day to maintain healthy bone density. There is no need for supplementation as long as you eat a well-balanced diet, as the table below demonstrates.

Food	Portion size	Amount of magnesium
Broccoli	1 spear	32mg
Spinach (uncooked)	30g	34mg
Lentils	30g	73mg
Pumpkin seeds	28g	82mg
Cashews	28g	82mg
Porridge	100g	177mg

Brown rice, quinoa, wholegrains and Swiss chard are other good sources. On the other hand, alcohol may hinder the absorption of magnesium, and there is some evidence that refined sugar can do the same. Therefore, cutting down on the wine and sweets may be a simple way to boost magnesium levels.

Stomach acid, probiotics and absorption

As mentioned earlier, stomach acid plays a vital role in the digestive process. Yet levels naturally decline with age, with one estimate suggesting a 30 per cent reduction by the age of 60. This can have a significant impact on the body's ability to break down foodstuffs and absorb their nutrients, most notably calcium and magnesium. Therefore, one of the most serious consequences of low stomach acid can be osteoporosis, but it can also lead to cracked or weak fingernails, flatulence, undigested food in the stool and belching.

If you are diagnosed with low stomach acid, it may be worth trying a digestive enzyme supplement that contains hydrochloric acid (often listed as Hcl). These are available over the counter in health-food stores, but you should always consult your GP before taking them. In addition, they must only ever be taken with meals, as ingesting them at other times is not only pointless but can cause discomfort and maybe even a burning sensation. Remember, they contain acid.

Further along the digestive tract we find the gut bacteria – or microbiome – which has a multitude of roles. As we saw in Chapter 7, both prebiotics and probiotics can help to keep these beneficial bacteria healthy, which means they have the potential to enhance the absorption of minerals such as magnesium and calcium in the intestines. By way of a reminder, prebiotic foods provide fuel in the form of fermented fibre for existing gut bacteria. Some of the best sources are chicory, Jerusalem artichokes, leeks, garlic, onions, asparagus, oats and barley. Meanwhile, probiotics – such as yoghurt, sauerkraut, miso, kefir, pickles, kombucha and sourdough bread – are said to have similar health benefits, although through a different mechanism, because they themselves contain millions of beneficial bacteria and therefore cause an immediate increase in the number in the gut. Alternatively, if you don't like the idea of fermented foods, you could always take a probiotic supplement (see Chapter 16).

Exercise

Of course, all forms of regular exercise provide countless health benefits. However, when it comes to maintaining bone density, some activities may have little effect while others might even do more harm than good. For instance, so-called 'cardio' exercise, such as running, fast walking or aerobics, does little to promote bone health.

By contrast, weight-bearing exercise that pitches you against the force of gravity results in an increase of collagen when stress is placed on a bone, which in turn attracts extra mineral deposits, leading to enhanced bone density and strength. Sports such as basketball and volleyball, which involve a lot of jumping, are particularly good at promoting this. Alternatively, simply climbing stairs, skipping or doing push-ups can be beneficial, as can lifting dumb-bells or using a fixed machine with weights at the gym.

Meanwhile, it is advisable to avoid some of the more frenetic types of exercise and especially contact sports if you have poor bone density and therefore an increased risk of fracture. It might be worth investing in a few sessions with a personal trainer as they will set you on the right path and provide some pointers on how to get the maximum benefit from whatever activity you choose to do.

CHAPTER 10

Digestion and the gut

Vital influences on your health

O ver recent years, there has been a surge of interest in gut health – specifically in relation to helpful bacteria and yeast – with countless books and websites devoted to the subject. However, this is not a fad. Rather, as our understanding of the synergistic relationship between gut bacteria and human well-being deepens, it is becoming increasingly clear that this immensely complex topic has wide-reaching implications for general and particularly digestive health.

More than one thousand different species of bacteria may reside in the human gut, although each of us has our own unique configuration involving more of some and fewer of others. The majority are classified as either bacteriodetes or firmicutes, and the ratio between these two types is particularly important. While we hear a lot about 'good' gut bacteria, there are plenty of 'bad' ones, too. By and large, though, good gut health is a simple matter of maintaining an optimum number of the beneficial bacteria, as they are able to crowd out most of the less favourable varieties.

The number and type of gut bacteria are established at birth, but thereafter the proportions fluctuate incessantly. For instance, countless factors, such as medications, supplements and diet, will have had a profound impact on the proportions and amounts of various species of bacteria in your gut.

The role of gut bacteria

Problems with gut bacteria have been linked to numerous health conditions, ranging from irritable bowel syndrome to food allergies and intolerance, loss of bone density, weight gain, loss of appetite, chronic fatigue, atherosclerosis, inflammation, arthritis and other autoimmune diseases. They also have a significant impact on mood (often referred to as the gut/brain axis) and may even be a factor in depression.

By now, I hope you appreciate the importance of fibre in the diet. In the gut, friendly bacteria produce short-chain fatty acids (SCFAs) from this fibre, which the cells that line the intestines then use as fuel. These cells have many roles, including the regulation of blood glucose, so it could be said that gut bacteria play an indirect but crucial role in appetite and weight management.

As this example indicates, eating gut-friendly foods and boosting your corps of beneficial bacteria can promote general good health in some surprising ways. We have discussed these gut-friendly foods (which come in two forms – probiotics and prebiotics) in previous chapters, but now it's time to explore them in rather more detail.

Prebiotic foods

As we have seen, prebiotic foods contain indigestible fibre. This means that it passes through the stomach and into the first section of the gut – the small intestine – where it provides the fuel that beneficial bacteria need in order to flourish.

There are three major types of prebiotic fibre – inulins, oligosaccharides and arabinogalactans – all of which are polysaccharides. That is, they are carbohydrates that contain several sugar cells, bonded together in chains. You need a regular supply of all three to promote good gut health.

Among the best prebiotic foods are:

- Artichokes
- Carrots
- Radish
- Asparagus
- Onions
- Garlic
- Leeks
- Sweet potato
- Chicory
- Berries
- Apples
- Banana
- Mango
- Coconut flour
- Quinoa
- Chia seeds
- Pumpkin seeds
- Sesame seeds
- Wild rice

Probiotic foods

Many species of bacteria fall under the umbrella term 'probiotics', although most of them are members of either the *Lactobacillus* or the *Bifidobacterium* family, both of which are associated with a wide variety of health benefits.

All lactic acid bacteria, such as *Lactobacillus*, can be added to dairy products, which causes the milk to ferment, creating foodstuffs that have a probiotic effect. In addition, though, almost any carbohydrate-rich food, including vegetables, can be fermented using a combination of salt and sugar and/or *Lactobacillus* cultures known as starters. There are plenty of step-by-step instructions online and it's a surprisingly straightforward process. Alternatively, fermented vegetables are widely available in mainstream shops.

You might find the idea of fermented food unappetising, not to mention some of the terms that are linked to these products, such as 'fungus'. However, bear in mind that yoghurt is fermented, as are those staples of burger restaurants – gherkins – so you have probably been consuming probiotics for years without even knowing it.

Ideally, you should try to incorporate a range of fermented foods in your diet, because they all contain slightly different strains and combinations of bacteria with their own specific benefits.

Among the best probiotic foods are:

- Sauerkraut (shredded cabbage)
- Kimchi (shredded cabbage and other vegetables)
- Tempeh and natto (fermented soya beans)
- Miso (soya beans fermented with a fungus called koji)
- Kombucha (fermented tea)
- Gherkins (pickled cucumbers)
- Kefir (tart fermented milk)
- Yoghurt
- Cheddar cheese
- Gouda cheese
- Parmesan cheese

Alcohol and the gut

It is often assumed that alcohol has an entirely negative effect on the level of probiotics in the gut. Yet some research suggests that moderate drinkers actually have a wider variety of beneficial bacteria than non-drinkers. That said, excessive alcohol consumption certainly seems to reduce the concentration of several strains of *Lactobacillus* in the gut, with studies showing particularly poor levels among alcoholics. This may be one of the reasons why heavy drinkers are at increased risk of a range of health conditions that are linked to inflammation (see Chapter 7).

Recently, I have been wondering if the potentially harmful effects of drinking might be offset by eating probiotics at the same time. It seems logical that some sort of balance could be achieved, although I would certainly not advocate a diet that consisted of several glasses of Rioja accompanied by a large lump of Parmesan each night. While this might help to maintain your microbiome, it would be detrimental to your health in countless other ways. Therefore, as ever, my advice is to stick to the recommended maximum of fourteen units per week.

Sugar

While fat was vilified throughout the seventies and eighties, now it seems to be the turn of sugar. However, although it would be great to blame all of our health woes on a single culprit, nutrition is obviously much more nuanced and complicated than that.

In terms of sugar and the gut, it is now widely believed that a diet that is high in refined sugars encourages the growth of harmful bacteria at the expense of good bacteria. This may well be true, but it is difficult to establish a definitive link between high sugar intake and poor gut health. This is because people who eat a lot of refined sugar also tend to eat a lot of saturated fat and little dietary fibre, so their diets may be harmful to the probiotics in their guts for a variety of reasons.

That said, cutting down on sugar is certainly advisable. Most of us are well aware that an apple is a healthier option than a chocolate bar, as is an oatcake with some hummus rather than a handful of biscuits. But what about supposedly 'healthy' versions of what are usually considered guilty pleasures? For instance, the packaging of a box of brownies may boast that they contain 'no refined sugar' or only 'natural sugars'. In such products, granulated white sugar is often replaced with sugars sourced from dates, coconut or rice. However, don't be fooled: after ingestion, these so-called 'healthy' sugars behave in almost exactly the same way as the refined sugar you were trying to avoid. For instance, they will also tip the balance in favour of harmful rather than good bacteria in the gut. Moreover, several studies suggest that sweeteners made from fructose (fruit sugar) and syrups such as agave are no better.

The UK guidelines advise that no more than 5 per cent of your daily energy should come from 'free sugars', which equates to roughly 30g per day. A free sugar is one that is added to food, such as the white sugar in cakes, confectionery and fizzy drinks. By law, this must appear in the list of ingredients on the packaging, and the closer it is to the top, the more sugar the product contains, because the ingredients are listed by weight. The likes of honey, syrups (such as date, glucose and rice) and fruit juice also fall within this category.

In addition, a panel on the packaging should give precise details of the amounts of fat, protein and carbohydrates the product contains, with carbohydrates then subdivided into 'of which sugars'. If this figure exceeds 22.5g per 100g, then the product is considered to be a 'high sugar', while less than 5g per 100g is categorised as 'low sugar'. It goes without saying that high-sugar foods should be eaten infrequently or preferably not at all. As a guide, a can of cola has 39g of sugar, four fingers of a well-known chocolate bar 21.3g, a tube of wine gums has 15g and a brownie from a high-street coffee shop 38g. (Incidentally, a seemingly healthier option from the same establishment – a granola bar – is scarcely any better as it contains 30g.) Finally, every lump that is added to tea or coffee provides 1.5g of free sugar, which may seem a modest amount, but it soon adds up.

Fruit and fruit juices

Whenever a handful of fruit is passed through a juicer, almost all of the fibre is removed in the process of freeing up the liquid … and the sugars. You will remember that fibre slows down digestion, so eliminating it in this way means that the sugars the fruit contains are absorbed much more quickly than they would have been if it had been eaten in its natural, solid state. Therefore, a large glass of apple juice, drunk quickly, has the potential to overwhelm the body's sugar-processing system, resulting a steep blood glucose spike, whereas eating several whole apples does not. A smoothie – which involves blending rather than juicing the fruit – is something of a halfway house because, while the fibre is at least consumed, it is broken down (in effect, partially digested), so it has a limited capacity to delay the digestion process.

You may have seen press articles claiming that there is just as much sugar in a smoothie or fruit juice as there is in a can of cola. Now, it should be pointed out that these sugars are not the same, as fizzy drinks contain sucrose and glucose whereas the smoothies and juices contain fructose. Nevertheless, such scare stories do at least draw attention to the fact that fruit – especially in juice form – is not necessarily good for your health, especially when consumed in excessive amounts.

Of course, in its natural state, fruit is a very worthwhile source of both fibre and antioxidant nutrients. However, while the latter remain intact no matter how you consume your fruit, the former is completely lost if you juice it and rendered far less effective if you blend it into a smoothie. This is why you should only ever count fruit juice as one of your five a day, regardless of how many glasses you drink. Therefore, I recommend limiting yourself to just one, possibly at breakfast. In that case, you could combine it with, say, porridge, berries and nuts – a meal that contains protein, fibre and fat, all of which will help to slow the absorption of the juice's free sugars.

It may sound dull, but moderation in all things – even fruit juice – is usually the best way to go.

PART TWO

The ManFood plan

CHAPTER 11

Introducing the ManFood plan

N ow that we have explored nutrition in relation to ten crucial aspects of male health, it's time to put everything together. There's a lot of information in the pages that follow, because there's a huge range of nutrients to take into account when compiling an eating plan for optimum health.

Sometimes I get the sense of a strange divide between 'nutrition' and 'food', because it's possible to lose some of the joy of eating if we focus too much on what our food contains. I don't want you to look across a field on a summer's day, with the corn swaying in the breeze, and think nothing but 'fibre and vitamin C' or see only omega 3 and selenium in an aquarium of beautiful fish. This can become a problem, especially when diets adopt a deeply scientific approach, but please don't think that nutritionists aren't foodies. In fact, almost all of us love our food and enjoy eating.

The ManFood plan combines the pleasure, variety and flavours of tasty food with the nutritional science that will help you live a healthier life and reduce your risk of developing the conditions that we discussed in Part One of this book. Subsequent chapters provide far more detailed guidelines, but for now it may be useful to have a brief look at a typical breakfast and main course to see how the plan works in practice.

Let's say you start the day with a bowl of porridge, topped with walnuts, chopped apple and a dollop of natural, live yoghurt. In addition to the pleasure and satisfaction you'll get from this breakfast, it contains plenty of nutrients that will enhance your well-being:

- Oats: beta-glucan, other forms of fibre, copper, vitamin B1, magnesium, chromium and zinc.
- Walnuts: omega 3 (ALA), copper, protein, fibre, biotin, magnesium and potassium.
- Apple: polyphenols, fibre, ursolic acid and vitamin C.
- Yoghurt: calcium, probiotics, zinc and vitamins B2 and B12.

Specifically, these nutrients are beneficial to health in the following ways:

- Beta-glucan, other forms of fibre and omega 3 will help you to manage your cholesterol.
- Vitamins B12 and B2 and probiotics reduce homocysteine.
- Vitamin C and ursolic acid both have important roles to play in combating prostate enlargement and inflammation.
- Omega 3, fibre and vitamin C all contribute to cognitive function.
- B vitamins, copper, zinc and magnesium are involved in making energy and regulating the body's stress response.
- Magnesium and calcium are essential for good sleep, testosterone and bone health.
- Fibre, probiotics, protein, omega 3 and vitamin C help to reduce inflammation.
- Probiotics help to maintain bone density.

In addition, the combination of protein and fibre helps to maintain constant energy levels throughout the morning and should keep hunger at bay for several hours.

Finally, and crucially, this simple breakfast is easy to make and tastes great. Practicality is a key component of the ManFood plan, which is why it focuses on healthy food that you will want to eat over the long term. It's not all about kale smoothies and quinoa.

For instance, let's take a look at a typical ManFood main meal: grilled chicken breast with a baked sweet potato, cauliflower and mushrooms. This contains the following key nutrients:

- Chicken: vitamins B3, B5, B6 and B12, potassium, magnesium, zinc and selenium.
- Sweet potato: vitamins A, B1, B2, B3, B5 and B6, biotin, potassium, fibre and copper.
- Cauliflower: indole-3 carbinol, sulforphane, vitamins C, B1, B2, B3 and K, folate and fibre.
- Mushrooms: copper, selenium, vitamins B2, B3, B5 and D, fibre and potassium.

These nutrients provide the following benefits:

- Vitamins C and D, fibre, indole-3 carbinol and sulforphane are all required for good prostate health and aid cognitive function.
- Vitamin D, magnesium and zinc support testosterone production.
- Vitamin D is also crucial for good bone health.
- Copper, magnesium, zinc, B vitamins and biotin play important roles in the body's conversion of glucose into energy and the stress response.
- Fibre and antioxidants such as vitamin C, selenium, copper and carotenoids help combat inflammation and

support cognitive function. Fibre is also important for promoting good gut health.

In addition, the combination of protein from the chicken and fibre from the three other ingredients slows down digestion, which helps to keep glucose levels stable and regulates appetite.

Once again, this meal is easy to make and contains no exotic, unfamiliar or unpalatable ingredients, yet it offers a wide range of health benefits. Consequently, it ticks both of the main boxes of the ManFood plan.

In addition, I should point out that there is no need to follow the plan slavishly. It is perfectly feasible to chop and change ingredients to suit your personal tastes. For instance, in certain meals, you might want to exchange fish for poultry, or use lentils and beans in place of red meat. That's absolutely fine, but just make sure you always swap like with like: exchanging apples for cider or brown rice for French fries is clearly *not* acceptable.

Motivation

Over the course of many years of clinical practice, I have learned that most people – and especially men – are motivated by setting goals, especially if there are tangible benefits from achieving those goals.

Let's take a typical scenario. A routine blood test reveals that a middle-aged man's cholesterol is a little high, so his GP refers him to me for help with dietary changes. We work out a suitable plan together and he checks in every couple of weeks to confirm that he is following the advice. Three months pass, and at his next scheduled blood test his overall cholesterol has reduced and the ratio of HDL to LDL ('good' to 'bad' cholesterol) is more favourable.

In this case, a specific goal (reduce cholesterol), firm time-frame (the three months between blood tests) and impartial witness (the GP) provide a compelling, motivational combination for someone who responds well to goals and deadlines. Something similar may work equally well for you if your principal aim is to get your cholesterol under control, lose a particular amount of weight or decrease your risk of diabetes by reducing your average blood glucose level, because all of these involve meeting definitive targets.

On the other hand, finding the motivation to improve *general* health and well-being may be more difficult. We all find it hard to give up bad habits if there are no immediate, measurable, obvious benefits. And, indeed, it might be several years before the advantages of following the ManFood plan become apparent. However, rest assured, you will benefit from it in the long run, because it delivers the right balance of protein, fats and fibre-rich complex carbs as well as all of the nutrients you need for a healthy life. It's also easy to follow, flexible, convenient and, most importantly, tasty and satisfying.

In my experience, it's impossible to stick to overly prescriptive, strict diets and food plans for any length of time. You might follow them for a week or two, or even a couple of months, but eventually your motivation and willpower starts to fade and you succumb to temptation and fall off the wagon. Once that happens, you feel demoralised and find it extremely difficult to get back on.

The ManFood plan is very different because it comprises familiar, enjoyable foods and meals that you can mix and match to suit yourself, so it provides almost limitless flexibility as well as flavour.

Food allergies and intolerance

If you are living with a food allergy or intolerance, you are doubtless well versed in avoiding certain foods. Of course, you should continue to do this whenever a problematic food features in the ManFood plan. Simply ensure that you replace it with an alternative foodstuff with similar properties (for instance, soya rather than dairy yoghurt).

CHAPTER 12

Making smart food choices

The debate over which is the greater evil – carbs or fat – has been raging for fifty years now, and it shows no sign of abating. Throughout the seventies and eighties, the general consensus was that there was a direct link between fat and heart disease, not to mention obesity, so we were all told to adopt a low-fat diet. However, by the late 1990s, the blame had started to shift to carbohydrates, and specifically sugar. Consequently, millions of people around the world abandoned the old low-fat doctrine and embraced the Atkins diet – a very high-protein, low-carb plan – that Robert Atkins had first formulated in 1972.

However, low-carb diets date back even further than that. For instance, they became popular in the latter half of the nineteenth century after a formerly obese funeral director, William Banting, published a booklet called *Letter on Corpulence, Addressed to the Public* in 1863. Banting lost weight after limiting his diet to nothing but meat, vegetables, fruit and dry wine. The ensuing movement was so popular that his low-carb approach became known as 'Banting'.

Low- and no-carb plans tend to eschew grains and starch. In practice, this means no bread, pasta, potatoes, rice, noodles or sugar. The carbohydrates in vegetables are deemed acceptable, but fruit is sometimes excluded, too. Research into the effects of low-carb weight-loss plans has been extensive, and this has revealed that they do not outperform other restricted-calorie diets (low fat or otherwise) over the long term. Nevertheless, supporters of the low-carb lifestyle are vociferous and hold a deep conviction that many serious health issues – including dementia, depression and cardiovascular disease as well as obesity – can be traced back to excessive consumption of carbs.

You may have tried a low-carb diet in the past and may have experienced weight loss as well as a number of additional health benefits. However, it is probable that most – if not all – of those extra benefits were simple side-effects of losing the weight, rather than due to cutting out carbs. In addition, almost invariably, whenever I advise a client to make some changes to their diet, they embark on the new plan with gusto. At the beginning, they pay close attention to what they are eating and are far more mindful than previously, usually consuming fewer calories overall and/or favouring foods that are generally viewed as 'healthy'. In itself, this is likely to generate a variety of health benefits.

However, personal experience with clients and a host of independent research suggest that low-carb plans demand a huge amount of self-control and willpower, so they are unsustainable over the long term for most people. Perpetually avoiding all starchy carbs is incredibly difficult because they are everywhere, and sooner or later you are likely to give in and have a slice of birthday cake, a sandwich on a long train journey or some chips at a social event, if only because you don't want to appear rude by refusing. And once the low-carb spell has been broken, it's almost impossible to recapture that initial enthusiasm for the diet. You start to allow yourself a few more carbs here and there, then maybe some treats, such as the chocolate and biscuits you have avoided for months, and before you know it all of the weight you worked so hard to lose is back. Moreover, all too often, this weight gain is accompanied by a sense of disappointment and disillusionment, which can lead to comfort eating, so you end up in a worse situation than you were in the first place.

This is one of two main reasons why carbs are not excluded from the ManFood plan. The other is that many carb-rich foods are also excellent sources of highly beneficial dietary fibre. In short, a diet that incorporates a limited amount of carbs is more practical, more sustainable and even more healthy over the long term than one that eschews them altogether.

But what does a limited amount of carbs mean in practice? Well, here are some ideas:

- An open sandwich rather than a filling within two slices of bread.
- A tablespoon of pasta, rice, quinoa or millet as an accompaniment for main meals.
- A small teacup rather than a large bowl of porridge.
- Two or three new potatoes rather than a portion of chips with a main meal.
- A small baked potato with the fibre-rich skin left on.
- A couple of squares of chocolate rather than a whole bar.
- A palmful of rice noodles with a stir-fry.
- A tablespoon of basmati rice *or* a small portion of saag aloo with an Indian meal, not both.

As long as you are sensible and follow these rough guidelines, your body should get all the carbs it needs, which will make it easier to avoid sweets, baked goods and desserts.

CHAPTER 13

Breakfast

Your breakfast should be easy to make, appetising, provide consistent energy throughout the morning and, of course, contain many of the essential nutrients you need for optimum health. This may seem quite a tall order for such a small meal, but the ManFood plan takes all of these requirements into account to give you the best possible start to each day.

First and foremost, I recommend combining at least two food groups (in this case protein and complex carbohydrates), since this slows digestion, which in turn stabilises blood glucose, provides consistent energy, and suppresses appetite for longer. Then you should start looking for ways to give yourself an early-morning boost of nutrients.

The standard breakfast

When I was growing up in the 1970s, the standard breakfast was toast with jam or marmalade and/or sugary cereal out of a packet. Perhaps this is still the case for many of you today. While our northern European counterparts are partial to savoury breakfasts, for some reason we Brits have typically had a sweeter tooth, particularly first thing in the morning. However, this is one tradition that we should all try to break.

For instance, if you were to eat a piece of granary toast with a slice of ham or a dollop of hummus rather than jam as a topping, the addition of protein to the fibre-rich bread would make this a quite well-balanced breakfast in itself. Then, ideally, you might want to add a sliced tomato, as this is one of the best sources of two essential nutrients: lycopene and potassium.

Cereal can be healthy too, but in this case the type you choose and what you add to it make all the difference. Most cereal manufacturers shout about the high fibre content of their wholegrain products, but have you ever taken a close look at the list of ingredients? For instance, one famous wholegrain wheat biscuit contains two different added sugars. Or maybe you prefer good old-fashioned cornflakes? Unfortunately, they too have two forms of added sugar. Now, both of these products do indeed contain a reasonable amount of dietary fibre, and to some extent it offsets the sugar they contain, but sprinkling on an extra teaspoonful yourself will outweigh all of the benefits provided by the fibre. Therefore, perhaps add some low-sugar fruit and/or a source of protein instead.

Muesli may be a better option, but again you need to be careful as many brands contain much more sugar than you might expect, particularly when the dried fruits are dusted with free sugar. In addition, all of those sultanas, raisins and lumps of dried pineapple contain much higher concentrations of sugar than their fresh counterparts. In addition, even a generous bowlful may be surprisingly low in protein, because many manufacturers keep the nut content quite meagre in order to reduce costs. Therefore, if you like muesli, try to find one with no added sugar and have a small amount, say a teacup full and, if necessary, add a small handful of extra nuts to meet your protein requirements.

Granola is usually all carbs and sugar, so while it can be a useful addition to other breakfast foods, you should limit yourself to no more than half a teacup, perhaps mixed with fruits, nuts and yoghurt.

By contrast, eggs are a wonderful breakfast staple, not least because they are a great source of protein. These days, it's quite easy to find eggs from hens that have flaxseed added to their feed, which results in some omega 3 in the yolks. They are also naturally good sources of choline, which is required for transmission of signals between nerves, as well as vitamin D, which benefits prostate, sleep and testosterone health. A simple breakfast of a couple of boiled eggs with some complex carbs is a reasonable option, but lacks many of the nutrients that are found in fruits and vegetables. Therefore, it's a good idea to add avocado, spinach or tomato. You don't have to craft an Instagram-friendly plate: just mash the eggs into a bowl with any vegetable you like or half a small avocado. A slice of toast will provide the requisite amount of fibre, or crumble an oatcake on top. You might also add two generous teaspoons of seeds, such as a mixture of pumpkin and sesame, or three Brazil nuts, to provide protein, fibre and crunch along with selenium, which helps to maintain prostate health and supports cognitive function.

You can cook the eggs any way you like, although obviously poaching or boiling means no fat is involved, which keeps the calories down. (The eggs themselves are 11 per cent fat, so there's no need to add any more.) If you prefer your eggs fried, they should be cooked at a low temperature and not for too long. I fry mine in a little butter and cover the pan to reduce the cooking time. Scrambled eggs absorb all of the fat they are cooked in, so go easy on the butter or oil and, again, keep the temperature low.

Porridge can aid heart health and cognitive function, reduce inflammation and help with weight management, but only if you restrict yourself to a modest bowlful, rather than the huge portions that seem to be the norm. I recommend no more than a teacup-sized serving with a tablespoon of plain or Greek yoghurt stirred in for their probiotics (good for cardiovascular, inflammation, bones and gut) and calcium (bones). Add some walnuts for their omega 3 (cognitive function, inflammation and weight management), minerals (heart, sleep, stress, energy, testosterone and bones) and fibre (heart, cognitive function, weight management and inflammation) plus berries (prostate, cognitive function, heart, stress, energy and inflammation). As a guide for proportions, almost fill a teacup with the berries, then fill to the brim with the nuts, which will help to keep the calories in check.

A typical full English contains all of the food groups and plenty of nutrients, but usually far too much fat and 850 calories or more (i.e. a more than a third of the recommended maximum intake). If you really cannot resist, try ordering a half English, add no butter to the toast (which should be granary or wholemeal to increase the fibre) and opt for poached rather than fried or scrambled eggs. Even then, this should be a very occasional treat, rather than a daily routine.

Milk and alternatives

Back in the seventies, there were only two choices when it came to milk: skimmed or full fat. You may remember the milkman leaving bottles with either red or gold tops, with the latter signifying full fat. Robins and sparrows soon worked out the difference, as they would peck through the gold tops to get at the cream but leave the red tops alone. Now we also have semi-skimmed, 1 per cent (halfway between skimmed and semi-skimmed) and lactose free, as well as coconut, nut and soya milks. The range of choice is wonderful, especially if you are on a restricted diet, although I wonder what the birds would make of them if they were all left on the doorstep.

If you are a traditionalist and prefer cow's milk, then you should know that full fat contains 3.6 per cent fat, semi-skimmed 1.8 per cent and skimmed less than 0.3 per cent. In terms of energy, this means that a 250ml glass of skimmed milk contains 83 calories while full fat has 115, so there's not much difference. Therefore, if you think skimmed milk tastes like white water, it's fine to stick with full fat or semi-skimmed. All three types contain an easily absorbed form of calcium, a little vitamin D and B12, and some potassium.

Soya milk is worth considering as it has roughly the same amounts of protein, carbs and calories as cow's milk. In addition it contains isoflavones (which play an important role in prostate health; see Chapter 2) and is often fortified with extra calcium and vitamin D. However, steer clear of any brands that add sugar as this will cause an almost immediate increase in blood glucose as it is not bound to fibre.

Nut milks are made by blending nuts with water and then extracting the pulp. The resulting liquid is sometimes marketed as 'mylk'. Most of these products are good sources of B vitamins and vitamin E as well as several essential minerals, including magnesium, calcium, zinc, selenium and potassium, in varying proportions, depending on which nut is used.

Both nut and soya milks are also used to make yoghurts that provide all of the same nutrients. Once again, though, check the label carefully as even those that are categorised as 'plain' may have added sugar. (The most popular brand has 2g of added sugar per 100g.)

Coconut milk and yoghurt are becoming increasingly popular, even though they contain quite a lot of saturated fat. For instance, a 100ml serving of coconut milk has 2g of saturated fat, while a 250ml pot of coconut yoghurt contains 20g. The latter is equivalent to the recommended daily allowance in just one quite small dessert.

In Chapter 2, I recommended a maximum of four modest servings of dairy products each day as any more may result in excess calcium (which can be harmful to the prostate) and over-production of insulin growth factor (which may increase the risk of cancer). So, you could have some dairy with breakfast, a few splashes of milk in tea and coffee throughout the day, maybe a yoghurt with your lunch and some cheese and crackers in the evening. Just remain mindful of those four servings. If you feel that you are regularly exceeding this limit, it might be an idea to use nut or soya products in place of traditional dairy from time to time. This is becoming increasingly easy to do, not least because most coffee shops now stock a wide variety of milks. Incidentally, a typical coffee-shop latté contains around 250ml of milk, a flat white a little less and a cappuccino around 170ml. In old money, this means that a single coffee often contains half a pint of milk – something that would have been unthinkable to our grandparents' generation.

When to eat breakfast

Many people skip breakfast altogether, or just nibble something very small, often because they feel they don't have the time to prepare and eat a more substantial meal. Instead, they tend to grab a sugary snack and a milky coffee on the way to work.

It will probably come as no surprise to hear that it is much better to opt for something a bit healthier. This does not need to be anything fancy, or even freshly prepared. A small bowl of leftovers from yesterday's lunch or dinner will do just fine, as will a slice of ham and an oatcake (you don't even have to eat them together), an apple and a couple of Brazil nuts, or a small pot of plain yoghurt followed by a banana a few minutes later as you cycle or drive to the office or board the train. Alternatively, you could hard boil an egg the night before and eat it with an oatcake or rye cracker.

It's more difficult to find a healthy, well-balanced breakfast on the morning commute, but if you feel you must leave the house with an empty stomach, the usual guidelines apply: ensure that you eat a combination of all the main food groups (including protein and fibre), keep added sugar to a minimum and, if possible, try to get some essential vitamin and minerals, too. See the Food on the Go section in Chapter 15 for some options that are rather more healthy than a chocolate bar and a croissant.

Breakfast options

Option 1: Eggs

- Boiled
- Scrambled
- Poached
- Fried
- Omelettes
- Frittatas

Then add a vegetable, ideally one or more of the following (although any vegetable will do):

- Asparagus
- Broccoli
- Mushrooms
- Green beans
- Peppers
- Spinach
- Tomato
- Kale
- Chard
- Cress
- Onions
- Leeks

In itself, this can be a healthy breakfast, although you would need a substantial serving of vegetables to get the optimum amount of fibre. For this reason, it can be a good idea to add some sort of grain, such as a heaped tablespoon of cooked brown rice or quinoa to scrambled eggs, an omelette or a frittata. Alternatively, how about a couple of boiled eggs and soldiers, made from toasted granary or wholemeal bread? Personally, I like to crumble an oatcake onto my eggs, regardless of how they are cooked, or use them instead of wheat-based soldiers.

Option 2: Porridge and yoghurt

You can make porridge with any milk you like, or just water, if you prefer. As for yoghurt, I suggest no more than three-quarters of a teacup. Again, you can use cow's milk yoghurt or any of the alternatives. Note that instant oats also contain fibre, but avoid the brands with added sugar.

Then add some fruit, such as:

- Orange
- Peach
- Apricot
- Cherries
- Melon
- Blackcurrants
- Kiwi
- Berries
- Apple
- Mango
- Banana
- Plum
- Guava
- Watermelon

While milk and yoghurt are both quite good sources of protein, I recommend adding some nuts and seeds for a little extra, especially as they will also boost the fibre, mineral and vitamin content of the meal. Try a combination of the following to suit your individual taste:

- Almonds
- Brazil nuts
- Cashews
- Sesame seeds
- Pumpkin seeds
- Walnuts

- Flaxseeds (linseeds)
- Chia
- Hazelnuts
- Hemp seeds
- Pecans
- Sunflower seeds

To make them more interesting, spread the seeds and nuts on a baking tray and gently toast them for ten to fifteen minutes at no more than 130°C/250°F/Gas Mark ½. Give them a stir halfway through and let them cool for at least thirty minutes before use. These toasted nuts and seeds have far more flavour and a crunchier texture than the raw versions. Just make sure you don't overcook them or use too high a heat. They can be stored in an airtight jar or box, where the addition of a vanilla pod will provide some extra flavour. (This also works well for raw nuts and seeds.)

Finally, a pinch of matcha powder on top of porridge or yoghurt is always a good idea, because matcha (a concentrated form of green tea) is especially rich in polyphenols. Alternatively, you could add a pinch of cocoa powder, as this is also a good source of the same nutrients.

Option 3: Cereals

Wholegrains are best, and make sure the brand you choose has little or ideally no added sugar. Check the detailed list of ingredients rather than the basic nutrition label, and remember that sugars are often listed as 'syrup' as well as 'sugar'.

Now add milk or yoghurt, nuts and fruit, as in Option 2. As for portion size, a single wholewheat biscuit is 18.5g, which amounts to a satisfying, relatively healthy breakfast once the extras have been added. There is no need to eat three to prove your manliness!

Option 4: Bread

As mentioned in Option 1, toast can be a useful addition to eggs-based breakfasts. However, if bread forms the main part of your first meal of the day, then the type you choose and what you have as an accompaniment are key.

Ideally, you should always plump for fibre-rich over low fibre. For guidance, I have listed all of the main types of bread in order of the amount of fibre they contain:

- High bran
- Multigrain
- Seeded
- Wholemeal
- Rye
- Granary
- White

A slice of white bread contains only around 1.5g of fibre, compared to 4.5g or more in the high-fibre options.

If you like your bread toasted and spread it with butter, it's easy to use far too much, because the butter melts into the toast. This might result in you getting close to your daily allowance of saturated fat – and eating too many calories – before you've even finished the first meal of the day. Therefore, you may want to consider some healthier options.

Ideally, your topping or spread should contain some protein, as this will slow down the digestion of the carbs in the bread, providing a steady supply of energy throughout the morning, rather than a sudden but short-lived burst. All of the following are good alternatives to traditional butter:

- Nut butter
- Ham
- Hummus
- Salmon or smoked salmon*
- Tuna*
- Mackerel*

- Sardines*
- Herring*
- Cheese**
- Avocado
- Chopped liver
- Bean pâté
- Baked beans

* Cooked fish can be used as a toast topping straight out of the tin, or mash it up with two tablespoons of lemon juice and a teaspoon of Greek yoghurt to make a paste.
** Limit yourself to a 28–30g portion of cheese (a block about the size of a small matchbox).

Your breakfast will contain much less protein, insufficient fibre and too much sugar if you choose jam or some other sweetened spread in place of any of these toppings. Such an option is not only less healthy over the long term but likely to result in low energy and hunger pangs within a couple of hours.

GLUTEN

Gluten is a type of protein that is found in wheat, barley and rye. Severe intolerance to gluten affects the lining of the intestines, reducing the body's ability to absorb nutrients. Known as coeliac disease, it affects around 1 per cent of the UK population. Symptoms include diarrhoea, constipation, mouth ulcers, flatulence, anaemia, bloating, fatigue and stomach cramps. If left untreated, coeliac disease can increase the risk of developing other conditions, especially osteoporosis and neurological disorders.

Many coeliacs are diagnosed between the ages of 40 and

60, which could be explained by the fact that that there was little testing for the disease before the 1990s. You should consult your doctor if you feel you may be suffering from the condition and they will arrange a thorough blood test. I strongly advise against the heavily advertised home-testing kits.

If the test reveals coeliac disease, your GP will advise you to avoid gluten altogether by eating grains such as rice and oats, rather than wheat. Many gluten-free breads, flours and baked goods are now available, and they contain almost exactly the same nutrients as standard bread – only the gluten is removed.

Breakfast drinks

If you enjoy a cup of tea or coffee first thing in the morning, you should be aware that a single teaspoon of sugar or honey will add about 6g of free sugar to the meal. You should watch your dairy intake, too, especially if you are partial to lattés or flat whites.

Green and matcha tea are better options as they are rich in polyphenols and catechins (see Chapter 2). In addition, be aware that matcha contains more caffeine than traditional black tea. On the other hand, if you are trying to limit your caffeine intake, you could try one of the many herbal teas instead.

A small (150ml) glass of fruit juice counts as one of your five a day and it boasts all of the polyphenols, carotenoids and other nutrients that are found in the whole fruit, but you should limit yourself to just one glass not only at breakfast but throughout the whole day. Any more will result in overconsumption of free sugar with none of the beneficial fibre that whole fruit contains.

CHAPTER 14

Main meals and snacks

The phrase 'a meat and two veg kind of guy' is often used to describe a man with an unsophisticated, no-nonsense, old-fashioned attitude to life. However, by now, you probably realise that a serving of meat and two different kinds of vegetables is not too bad at all in terms of providing all the nutrients you need.

Many people who contemplate adopting a healthier lifestyle are put off by the assumption that nutritious meals demand a great deal of preparation and culinary skill. But that assumption could not be more wrong. I'll show you how to produce meals that are tasty and interesting, include all of the major food groups and contain dozens of beneficial nutrients. And they are all easy to prepare, once you know how.

The basics

Let's start with the food groups. Very few foodstuffs contain nothing but fat or protein or carbs, so I have grouped them according to whichever element is most abundant.

As we saw throughout Part One, it is always advisable to combine all of the food groups at each meal (and even when snacking). Fibre, when eaten with protein, breaks down slowly, which helps keep you satisfied for longer. Ideally, you should aim to eat a little fat too, perhaps in the form of a dressing or a little olive oil on vegetables, although you will often not need to add any as many foods contain at least some fat.

When eating meat, trim off any visible white fat, and don't let the remaining fat brown too much. Poultry skin has long been vilified, even though it contains exactly the same beneficial nutrient – oleic acid – that is found in olive oil. Nevertheless, don't eat too much of it because it is also a significant source of calories.

As for fish skin, opinion is divided over whether to eat it. Although it contains some nutrients, it is also quite fatty, which is why it crisps up when seared or hot grilled. My feeling is that crispy skin is delicious, while the limp, soft skin of steamed or poached fish is rather unpleasant. If you agree, perhaps eat some (but not all) of the crispy skin when you grill your fish and discard the soft skin when you poach it.

The protein source of a main meal can be anything from poultry, meat or fish to tofu or beans. However, bear in mind that the UK Department of Health recommends eating no more than 70g of red meat each day. Meat is always a good source of iron (for energy), vitamin B12 (energy and heart) and protein, but the rest of the nutritional profile depends on what the animal has been fed. You may have heard of 'grass-fed' meat, which can have higher concentrations of a number of nutrients, including four times as much omega 3 as meat from grain-fed animals. However, it is also much more expensive and so may not be the most practical choice, especially as there are even better dietary sources of omega 3.

I suggest eating no more than 90g (cooked weight) of red meat a maximum of four times a week (although less would be preferable). For guidance, 90g of meat equates to three small slices, each of which is about the size of half a slice of bread.

Processed meats contain sodium nitrate, a preservative that is converted into nitrites on contact with saliva or other enzymes further along the digestive tract. These nitrites are then converted into nitric oxide or nitrosamine: the former is beneficial as it helps to reduce blood pressure (see Chapter 1), whereas the latter has been linked to colorectal cancer. Nitrosamine is also created when nitrites are combined with amino acids (the building blocks of protein) and heat. In other words, when you eat cooked and preserved meat, the level of nitrosamine in your body inevitably increases. Therefore, it is advisable to limit your intake of processed meat products, in terms of both amount and frequency. For reference, a slice of ham, a rasher of bacon or a sausage weighs around 30g, and research suggests that there is a small but significant increase in the risk of colorectal cancer if you exceed the recommended upper limit of 50g of processed meat per day.

Also note that the aforementioned 90g limit no more than four times a week encompasses *all* meat products – fresh, processed, grass-fed or whatever. So, if you hit your limit of 50g of processed meat by eating a couple of rashers of bacon for lunch, you should limit yourself to a maximum of 40g of steak or lamb at dinner. Better still, leave the red meat in the fridge for another day and choose something else instead.

Finally, we turn to complex carbohydrates, which differ from simple carbs in that they contain more fibre because they have not been refined or overly processed. You may be sick of hearing about fibre by now, but it's the bedrock of good nutrition, and in the ManFood context it plays a crucial role in maintaining good cardiovascular health and cognitive function, keeping weight under control, providing consistent energy, reducing inflammation and ensuring your digestive system remains in tip-top shape. Most of the UK population get about 18g of fibre per day, but ideally we should all be eating at least 30g to reap its many benefits.

Complex carbs are found in all grains, fruits, vegetables, beans (otherwise known as pulses or legumes) and tubers, although some contain fewer sugars and more fibre than others. If you include plenty of lightly cooked vegetables (so they retain some crunch) in your diet, you can get by without eating any grains at all, although the latter are an easy way to boost fibre intake for most people. For guidance, 100g of cooked broccoli contains 3.3g of fibre, whereas the same quantity of cooked brown rice has 1.8g, quinoa 2.8g and spinach 2.4g. So vegetables do indeed make fine sources of fibre.

Vegetables are also great sources of potassium (good for the heart), carotenoids (prostate, cognitive function), antioxidant vitamins (inflammation, heart, cognitive function), zinc (energy) and magnesium (sleep, prostate, stress, energy). In addition, bitter vegetables – such as Brussels sprouts, kale and cauliflower – contain indole-3 carbinol and sulforphane.

Much of the fibre in tubers is found in the skins. For example, 100g of mashed potato has 1.3g fibre, which isn't much, given the size of the portion, whereas a 100g baked potato, including the skin, contains more than double that amount – 2.9g. I am not suggesting that you should never eat mashed potato, but possibly think of it as an occasional treat, and always try to combine it with one of the more fibre-rich vegetables.

Putting everything together

Every meal should contain a little protein, some complex carbs and vegetables as this combination will give you consistent energy and should help with weight management. In other words, a dinner of steak and vegetables is healthy and well balanced, whereas steak and pasta with no vegetables is not.

No food is 100 per cent protein, although some contain much more than others, with animal products having the highest concentrations in addition to varying amounts of fat. Non-animal foods that are categorised as protein-rich, such as chickpeas, kidney beans and lentils, also contain relatively high levels of carbohydrates as well as fibre. Therefore, ideally, your diet should include at least some plant-based protein, and if you can manage to eliminate all animal-based protein from at least three meals a week, all the better.

That said, favouring specific foods that you do not particularly enjoy simply because they contain a little more protein can lead to a limited, repetitive, boring diet that you will find difficult to maintain. It is for this reason that the ManFood plan is built on variety. There's certainly no need to think that you must have a portion of lentils with every meal. The list of good sources of protein is almost endless, so there is plenty of scope to cherry-pick those that you find especially appealing, then mix them up to keep your diet interesting.

Below, I have compiled lists of all of the foods that enjoy the ManFood plan seal of approval. Simply observe the guidelines regarding food combinations, portion sizes and weekly limits and you will soon be well on your way to a healthier diet.

Poultry

- Chicken
- Turkey
- Quail
- Game hen
- Goose
- Partridge
- Guinea fowl
- Pheasant

Red meat

- Beef
- Veal
- Lamb
- Mutton
- Venison
- Liver (all types)
- Pork
- Ostrich
- Bison

Dairy and eggs

- All yoghurts
- All cheeses
- Milk (cow's, goat's and sheep's)
- All eggs

Fish

- Anchovies*
- Herring*
- Carp*
- Mackerel*
- Whitebait*
- Trout*
- Sardine*
- Salmon*
- Cod
- Eel
- Pollock
- Tuna
- Dab
- Flounder
- Swordfish
- Red snapper
- Monkfish
- Turbot
- Mullet
- Plaice
- Halibut

* Oily fish that contain high concentrations of the omega 3 fats DHA and EPA. The others are white fish that are lower in fat.

Other seafood

- Squid*
- Mussels*
- Oysters*
- Crab*
- Scallops
- Prawns
- Cockles
- Langoustines
- Lobster
- Octopus

* Contain small amounts of omega 3 fats.

Current NHS guidelines recommend eating at least one 140g portion of fish or other seafood each week. However, oily fish contain pollutants that may accumulate in the human body, so you should limit yourself to a maximum of four portions per week. Any other seafood that contains omega 3 – such as oysters and mussels – should also be included in this limit.

White fish may be enjoyed more often, with the exception of halibut, turbot, sea bass and sea bream, as they contain small amounts of omega 3. Therefore, they should be limited, though not avoided.

Beans (legumes and pulses)

- Cannellini beans
- Kidney beans
- Black beans
- Broad beans
- Butter beans
- Lentils (all varieties)
- Chickpeas
- Soya beans (and tofu)
- Black-eye peas
- Split peas
- Green peas
- Mangetout
- Peanuts

All beans contain complex carbohydrates and a healthy amount of fibre, as well as protein.

Nuts and seeds

- Pumpkin seeds
- Sesame seeds
- Sunflower seeds
- Almonds
- Pistachios
- Cashews
- Walnuts
- Brazil nuts
- Pecans
- Macadamias
- Hazelnuts
- Pine nuts

All nuts and seeds are good sources of protein and fibre, but they also contain saturated fat and omega 6 (which can increase inflammation). Walnuts are the exception to this rule, as they contain omega 3 in the form of ALA, rather than omega 6. Nevertheless, all nuts and seeds, including walnuts, should be eaten in moderation, perhaps sprinkled over salads, soups and vegetables, or a small handful as a snack.

Vegetables

- Asparagus
- Spinach
- Mushrooms
- Swiss chard
- Lettuce (all varieties)
- Peppers (capsicums)
- Kale
- Brussels sprouts
- Broccoli
- Cauliflower
- Rocket
- Watercress
- Pak choi
- Cabbage (all varieties and colours)
- Celery
- Onions (all varieties)
- Cucumber
- Romanesco
- Artichoke
- Swede
- Celeriac
- Leeks
- Spring greens
- Bean sprouts
- Garlic
- Tomato*
- Avocado*
- Seaweed
- Chilli peppers
- Courgette
- Green beans
- Aubergine
- Runner beans
- Radish
- Beetroot**
- Carrots**
- Pumpkin**
- Squash (all varieties)**
- Peas**
- Potato**
- Sweet potato**
- Corn**
- Yams**
- Parsnips**

* Although technically fruits, avocados and tomatoes are often viewed as vegetables, so I am happy to treat them as such. In addition to carbs, avocado contains some protein and monounsaturated fats.

** These vegetables all contain large amounts of starch, so in the ManFood plan they are treated as both a vegetable and a carb. I recommend limiting yourself to one small portion no more than five times a week. Green vegetables contain fewer carbs, and you should aim for three or four portions a day (yes – that says *day*).

Grains

- Quinoa
- Teff
- Wholewheat pasta
- Millet
- Couscous
- Egg noodles
- Bulgar
- Rice (wild, brown, white, red or bran)

Grains are mostly carbohydrate, so while they provide a little protein to your meal, they should not be considered a protein-rich food.

Building a meal

It bears repeating that the ideal combination for any meal, not least because it helps to keep blood glucose relatively stable, is some protein, some carbs and a large portion of vegetables. (Equally, you could eliminate the carbs and just have the protein and the vegetables.) Below, I suggest some simple, practical, tasty meal ideas, all of which follow this basic rule.

Starters

Of course, you could always skip the starter and just go straight for the main course, but something beforehand can be a convenient way to get some extra nutrients . . . and it can taste great, too. For instance, how about a bowl of vegetable soup? That could provide one or even two of the recommended five servings of fruit and vegetables a day.

Starters also provide useful opportunities to include fermented foodstuffs whose strong flavours might overwhelm the ingredients in a main course. Miso soup, rocket with Parmesan, and sauerkraut with a little cream cheese on a rye cracker all fall into this category. You can be as inventive as you like.

If you prefer a milder flavour, try a plate of sliced tomato, avocado and mozzarella cheese. Or smoked salmon (for the omega 3) on mini-toasts and/or with salad leaves and diced vegetables, such as radish and onion.

One final point: if you do choose to have a starter, you should bear in mind that you may need to reduce the size of your main dish, so that your total calorie intake is taken into account.

Now it's time to turn to those main courses.

Chicken

Given the range of delicious, healthy alternatives, you will soon find it easy to make a better choice than a bucket of chicken wings or a stuffed-crust pizza.

For instance, how about a chicken breast, cut into slices, served with a large salad consisting of lettuce, peppers, radish, celery, cucumber and tomato? You could have a slice of rye bread as an accompaniment, or add a tablespoon of cooked brown rice or quinoa to the salad as well as a few anchovies, if you like. Or perhaps use the same ingredients to make an open chicken sandwich.

You could bake a chicken fillet with turmeric, ginger and garlic and serve with curried vegetables and a generous tablespoon of rice, or half of a naan bread. Or rub the chicken with paprika and chilli powder, grill, and enjoy with a small baked potato and steamed vegetables. Alternatively, you could stir-fry the chicken with vegetables in a little walnut oil and serve with rice noodles or brown rice.

If you like casseroles, chicken with a few diced potatoes and a combination of herbs and spices makes a delicious evening meal, and any leftovers can be eaten for lunch the following day. Or you could slow-bake the chicken with cherry tomatoes and garlic cloves, then rinse the contents of a can of unsalted cannellini or mixed beans and stir them in for the last five minutes, giving them another stir after a couple of minutes. Top with fresh basil before serving.

Barbecued chicken and grilled corn is a smoky treat, best accompanied with a small baked potato and some ratatouille, which contains plenty of easily absorbed lycopene on account of the cooked tomatoes. If you have any leftovers after the barbecue, make any variety of vegetable soup, although use only a little potato (or other starchy vegetable) to thicken. Rinse a can of beans and stir into the soup a few minutes before serving, then place the charred chicken on top. (See the box below for advice on safe and healthy barbecuing.)

Chicken tacos or fajitas always benefit from the addition of a few beans and sliced vegetables to balance the starch and protein. Chicken risotto is fine, but most people use far too much rice in relation to the chicken, so watch that ratio and include a vegetable-based starter to ensure you cover all the food bases. Similar care should be taken with chicken pasta. Serve with a crunchy salad or stir spinach into the dish and include another serving of vegetables on the side.

For a vegetarian option, tofu, beans or lentils can be substituted for the chicken in many of these dishes.

BARBECUES AND CHARRED FOOD

Back in the day, in many households, the traditional summer barbecue was one of the few occasions when the man of the house cooked anything, and barbecuing still retains something of a macho image.

Most people agree that barbecued food tastes delicious, but charring red meat, poultry or fish over an open flame can produce two potentially carcinogenic substances – heterocyclic aromatic amines (HAA) and polycyclicaromatic hydrocarbons (PAH). So, although the UK climate usually ensures that open-air cooking is a fairly infrequent event in this country, it is still advisable to follow some simple rules when you do have an opportunity to enjoy a barbecue:

1. It is a good idea to cook food on the side of the grill, rather than in the middle, as this means it is not exposed to the hottest charcoal.
2. Raise the grill so that when fat drops on the coals, the flames don't come into contact with the food.
3. Marinating meat, fish and poultry before popping them on the grill can reduce the likelihood of burning or charring.
4. Do not start cooking until the flames have died down and the charcoal is merely glowing, as this will result in less smoke and lower flames.

→

In addition, basic hygiene rules are often overlooked during barbecues, which can result in food poisoning. For instance, raw meat is often left out of the fridge for hours while everyone waits for the flames to die down. Then, when cooking does finally get under way, the meat is often cooked at far too high a temperature, leaving it charred on the outside and raw in the middle. Finally, one set of tongs may be used to transfer the raw meat to the grill and then serve the cooked food to the guests. This makes them the perfect breeding ground for the likes of salmonella and E. coli.

Therefore, if you want to make al fresco dining memorable for the right reasons:

1. Use one set of tongs for raw meat and another for cooked food.
2. Keep the meat, fish and chicken in the fridge for as long as possible before cooking.
3. Let the coals warm through until they have an orange glow. Nevertheless, fat will inevitably drip onto them, causing flames, so move the food around to reduce its exposure to direct heat.
4. Consider microwaving the meat for a couple of minutes before placing it on the grill. Microwaves cook from the inside, so they are ideal for counteracting the problem of food that is raw in the middle. Alternatively, par-cook in an oven at a low temperature, then use the barbecue to complete the cooking process. Either of these methods will ensure that the food is safe but still has that delicious smoky flavour.

Steak

As mentioned earlier, the recommended maximum portion size for red meat is 90g when cooked (equivalent to about 100g raw) and you should limit yourself to no more than four portions per week. In addition, as always, it is advisable to combine this protein-rich food with a large serving of green vegetables and a small amount of starchy carbs if you want.

For instance, steak may be grilled and served with quinoa, steamed broccoli, spinach and diced squash, baked in a little olive oil and sprinkled with chilli powder and/or hot paprika. Or it could be sliced and stir-fried with shredded cabbage and bean sprouts, then served on a bed of rice or egg noodles. If you have previously used bottled sauces to add flavour, you should be aware that they are usually sources of sugar and saturated fat, not to mention monosodium glutamate. They are also unnecessary, as you can often replicate the flavours with fresh and dried herbs, nut or seed oil (such as walnut or sesame) and soy sauce.

Cooked steak is also delicious eaten cold in a sandwich, roll or pitta bread with lots of crunchy salad. Or how about barbecued and served with a small baked potato, grilled peppers and grilled onions?

Just remember to observe that limit of 90g, four times a week.

Fish

You will recall that a similar limit applies if you are partial to oily fish, although the portion size is larger – a maximum of four 140g servings each week. As long as you adhere to that rule, the benefits of eating protein-rich, omega-3-rich fish are undeniable, especially if you combine it with plenty of fresh vegetables. I have suggested salmon for all the dishes below, but any oily fish would serve equally well.

Try poaching a salmon and serve hot with spinach, courgettes and a little polenta. Or how about leaving the fish to cool and accompanying it with three or four new potatoes, coleslaw and cherry tomatoes? Alternatively, mash it up with a little avocado, a teaspoon of Greek yoghurt and a pinch of turmeric and spread on a slice of rye bread with a large green salad on the side.

Blackened salmon – which entails coating the fish with melted butter, Cajun spices or mixed Mediterranean herbs before searing – served with a side of wholewheat pasta in a tomato sauce, fresh broad beans and green peas is especially tasty. Or maybe you would prefer a broth packed with plenty of vegetables (such as pak choi, sliced carrot and wilted spinach) and a few rice noodles alongside stir-fried salmon, with sliced ginger and coriander sitting on top. If you are not a fan of Asian cuisine, flaked salmon with a little cooked spaghetti and a large serving of ratatouille might be more appealing.

Roast salmon with a pistachio crust (crush pistachios then mix with breadcrumbs, a little olive oil, salt and pepper to make a paste and smear on the fish before cooking) is best served with kale and green beans. Alternatively, slow-bake the fish with preserved lemons, braised leeks and diced peppers and serve on a small bed of brown or wild rice.

HOW TO BOOST YOUR NUTRIENTS

- Tossing a teaspoon of raw or toasted seeds (sesame, pumpkin, sunflower, etc.) over vegetables adds texture, fibre, protein and nutrients, not to mentions flavour. Sprinkle over soups, salads and stir-fries, too.
- Crushed walnuts provide some omega 3 as well as fibre and crunch.

- Garlic is a powerful antifungal and antibacterial agent, and it can help to reduce LDL (the 'bad' cholesterol). It is even more potent when crushed and left for twenty minutes before use.
- If appropriate, stir a teaspoon of tomato paste into vegetables and soups as this is rich in lycopene (an antioxidant that is particularly beneficial for prostate health).
- Make a sauce for fish, vegetables and grains out of plain yoghurt, mixed seeds and chopped herbs (such as flat-leaf parsley, dill or coriander) for extra probiotics, fibre and protein.
- If using the leftovers from dinner for lunch the next day, liven them up with hot sauce or a fresh yoghurt-based dressing, if appropriate. If the portion is small, complement it with a mixed salad or maybe a sliced boiled egg and a tablespoon of mixed nuts/seeds. (See the box on page 175 for more leftovers ideas.)
- For dressings, a combination of extra-virgin olive oil, mustard powder and lemon juice is a good option (add lemon rind for extra punch). Alternatively, a simple dressing of walnut oil and a pinch of salt is delicious with fish and beans, whereas horseradish sauce, lemon juice and olive oil works well with meat and tubers. If you buy bottled sauces, remember to check the ingredients carefully, as they often contain unnecessary added sugar.

Vegetarian and vegan

In my experience, vegetarians – and especially vegans – tend to be better informed than the general population with regard to nutrition. Consequently, if you fall into either of these categories, the chances are that your diet already adheres quite closely to most of the ManFood principles.

Nevertheless, it can be difficult to get all the nutrients you need if you eschew meat and fish, and especially if your diet includes no animal products whatsoever. The following advice may help.

Calcium

As we saw in Chapter 9, men over the age of 55 need some 1200mg of calcium each and every day to maintain healthy bone mass. Many people automatically think of dairy products when discussing calcium, but it is also found in relatively high concentrations in dark green vegetables, beans, nuts and seeds. See the table on page 120 for precise amounts per serving.

Protein

It's easy for carnivores to get all the protein they need, but you may have to be a little more creative if you follow a vegan or a vegetarian diet. The trick is to mix it up.

A total of twenty-two amino acids may be found in protein foods. However, eight of these are more important than the others because the human body is able to link them in various combinations to make the remaining fourteen. Therefore, understandably, these eight core amino acids are known as 'essential'. If a food boasts all eight, then the protein it contains is termed 'complete', as the full complement of amino acids can be manufactured from it.

Animal proteins – such as meat, fish and poultry – are always complete, whereas some vegan or vegetarian sources are not (although the likes of chickpeas, quinoa, nuts and most beans are). Rather than worry about which foods are complete or incomplete, however, the best idea is simply to eat a wide variety of protein-rich vegetables, such as different beans, nuts, tofu, tempeh, soya products, lentils, grains and peas. That way, you are certain to get all eight of the essential amino acids your body needs.

Without this sort of variation in your diet, you run the risk of developing protein deficiency. You should consult your GP and/or a nutritional professional if you suffer any of the following symptoms:

- Fatigue
- Raised appetite and cravings for sugar
- Poor muscle tone
- Hair weak or falling out
- Ridges on the fingernails and/or toenails

Omega 3

Omega 3 fats play a multitude of roles, such as maintaining cognitive function and combating inflammation. There are three different forms of this so-called 'good' fat: alpha linolenic acid (ALA), which is found in some plants; eicosapentaenoic acid (EPA); and docosahexaenoic acid (DHA), which is found in marine fish. Many of the principal benefits of omega 3 are most closely associated with DHA, although ALA, which is suitable for vegan and vegetarian diets, is almost as useful.

The best sources are rapeseed and olive oil, walnuts, purslane (which is edible, even though it is often classified as a weed), chia, hemp and linseed. It is advisable for vegetarians and vegans to use some or all of these on a regular basis. An omega 3 supplement might be beneficial, too (see Chapter 16).

Vitamin D

As we saw in Part One, vitamin D is important for good prostate, testosterone and bone health, and it also promotes good sleep. This essential nutrient is generally lacking among all UK adults, but the level of deficiency can be especially acute among those who follow a vegetarian or vegan diet.

Fortified orange juice and nut milks may help to mitigate this problem, along with a diet that is rich in mushrooms and soya products. However, a supplement is probably the best and most convenient solution (see Chapter 16).

Vitamin B12

Vitamin B12 plays an important role in heart health, energy and regulating stress, among many other functions. In nature, it is only found in animal products, but it can be added to the likes of vegan cheese and milk products. Nevertheless, if you follow a vegan or vegetarian diet, it is advisable to take a vitamin B12 supplement (see Chapter 16 for appropriate dosages, etc.).

Meat-free dishes

Tofu (which is made from mashed soya beans) and mycoprotein (which is usually known by the brand name Quorn) are both excellent, protein-rich meat substitutes. Meanwhile, the likes of lentils and chickpeas provide a healthy combination of carbs and protein. Some grains, such as millet and quinoa, similarly offer a mixture of protein and carbs. In short, a meat-free diet can be just as varied as any other.

For instance, there's the Asian classic stir-fried tofu with rice noodles and vegetables. Or perhaps try a lentil curry in a tomato-based sauce, served with brown rice and cauliflower. Or maybe a broad bean risotto (plenty of beans and not too much rice), with roast tomato, green beans and flaked almonds.

Miso soup with tofu, pak choi, broccoli and watercress is a good option as it is a tasty source of beneficial probiotics, as is sauerkraut on toasted ciabatta rubbed with garlic. The same is true of tempeh (fermented soya beans) with steamed rice and stir-fried vegetables, topped with a little sesame oil and soy sauce.

How about a simple dish of hummus with oatcakes (which also contain the beneficial fibre beta-glucan) and a green salad, or perhaps a hummus sandwich with sliced carrot, tomato and lettuce? If you prefer something warmer, many nut roasts also contain lentils, which makes them particularly rich sources of both protein and fibre. A simple mixed-bean casserole or stew, served over a baked sweet potato, is sure to keep hunger pangs at bay, too.

If you eat eggs and dairy products, then a frittata with as many diced vegetables as you can manage, along with a slice of bread, makes a satisfying meal. Or you could opt for a large salad with crunchy vegetables and some Cheddar cheese, topped with a poached egg (or walnuts may be used in place of the egg).

LEFTOVERS

Leftovers can often serve as the base for convenient and economical meals or snacks over subsequent days. Whether you have enough for a whole meal (say, an extra piece of fish or chicken) or just a couple of slices of tofu and a handful of vegetables, you can usually cobble together something quite tasty.

The trick with leftovers is to tweak them so you are not merely having a cold version of what you ate the night

→

before. A few herbs (fresh or dried) and a dash of dressing, such as hot sauce or nut oil, will enliven any leftover meal, while a spoonful of freshly cooked rice, quinoa or beans adds texture and complex carbs. (Remember that even leftover meals should contain protein, fibre, carbs and maybe a little fat.)

If I am left with a small portion of salmon fillet after finishing dinner, I will often mash it up with a drizzle of walnut or olive oil and half a teaspoon of sesame seeds for lunch the next day. This simple salmon paste is delicious with a handful of salad leaves or watercress and a couple of gherkins. Alternatively, add a couple of teaspoons of toasted pumpkin seeds, a pinch of cayenne pepper, some lemon juice and a splash of olive oil to the salmon and mash lightly with a fork, then serve with a generous tablespoon of wild or brown rice.

Beans can be a little bland, especially when cold, so I like to add a generous dash of hot sauce or some walnut oil along with a pinch of salt and pepper. Or you could warm a couple of tablespoons in a pan with toasted sesame oil, oregano, parsley and herbes de Provence, saffron, salt and pepper as an accompaniment for leftover salmon or chicken. An even easier option is to mix some stock (from a cube or a teaspoon of powder) with olive oil to make a sticky paste, then stir this into the beans before baking in a warm oven for fifteen minutes (stir every few minutes to stop the beans drying out).

A strongly flavoured oil, such as walnut or truffle, is often useful, as are strips of dried seaweed, as both can give leftovers that extra zing. By the same token, a tablespoon of Greek yoghurt or crème fraiche and lemon juice added to leftover beans, chilli, fish, meat or poultry can turn a humdrum meal into a delicious treat.

Simple meals

We all have busy lives, and sometimes we don't have the time or indeed the inclination to prepare an elaborate meal from scratch. With that in mind, I have compiled a list of simple dishes that require minimal effort. Most of them can be made from leftovers and/or foods that you probably already have in the cupboard or the fridge.

- Two hard-boiled eggs, mashed up with a small teaspoon of Greek yoghurt, half a diced red pepper and a pinch of curry powder, turmeric, black pepper and sea salt. Serve with salad leaves or spread on oatcakes or toast.
- Boil brown rice or quinoa in chicken or vegetable stock (simply add a stock cube to the water), allow to cool a little, place two tablespoons of the cooked rice on a plate, add a whole small can of sardines, tuna or salmon, then some radishes or celery for crunch.
- One tablespoon of hummus with carrots, celery and peppers on a rye cracker.
- Half a medium-sized avocado, tomato, mozzarella and a handful of spinach leaves. Dress with a two tablespoons of olive oil mixed with a drizzle of balsamic vinegar.
- Half a medium-sized avocado mashed with dried chilli flakes and sea salt, spread on a small piece of toast.
- Leftover (cold) green beans with crumbled feta cheese and salad leaves.
- Baked halloumi cheese served with sliced beetroot, lettuce and a dressing of horseradish sauce mixed with lemon juice and a little olive oil.
- Sliced leftover chicken served with diced spring onions, cos lettuce and two crumbled oatcakes.

- Cold Brussels sprouts mixed with two tablespoons of cooked and cooled quinoa (cook in stock) with a matchbox-sized portion of Parmesan cheese grated on top. Add some lemon zest for extra flavour.
- Baked potato with a third of the centre removed and replaced with baked beans. Top with a small amount of grated Cheddar cheese if desired.
- A slice of ham with a baked sweet potato, drizzled with walnut oil and topped with a large pinch of sunflower seeds.
- Two slices of smoked salmon served with a quarter of a medium avocado, lettuce and a slice of granary bread.
- Half a smoked mackerel with leftover roasted vegetables or salad leaves with a chopped raw carrot.
- Bowl of vegetable soup with half a can of rinsed butter beans mixed in. Drizzle a little nut oil on top and add a few crushed walnuts.
- Mixed-bean salad with tahini on oatcakes.
- One tablespoon of goat's cheese with cucumber, grated red cabbage and squash topped with toasted seeds served on an oatcake.
- Leftover roast beef, three cold new potatoes and kimchi.
- Tempeh served with cold rice and pickled vegetables.
- Ham and vegetable omelette.
- One drained and rinsed can of lentils warmed in a pan with a matchbox-sized block of Cheddar cheese cut into cubes and finely chopped flat-leaf parsley.
- Chicken breast and cherry tomatoes topped with torn basil leaves, olive oil and sea salt.
- One can of drained and rinsed cannellini beans mixed with cumin seeds, chilli powder and diced, cold, cooked potato.

- Cooked prawns mixed with cooked quinoa or rice, chopped celery, radish, dill and lemon juice, drizzled with extra-virgin olive oil.
- If you prefer a sandwich, use one slice of bread rather than two to keep the ratio of protein to starchy carbs well balanced. Then choose any protein source you like (meat, fish, tofu, beans, etc.) but remember to add some vegetables, such as tomato, lettuce or peppers.

SNACKS

The ManFood plan is nothing if not flexible, so it accommodates both the 'little and often' approach and 'three square meals a day'. Indeed, you could even chop and change between the two, perhaps snacking at weekends and sticking to set mealtimes during the working week. Either way is fine as long as you don't have three large meals *and* lots of snacks in the course of a single day.

Ideally, you should apply the basic principle of combining the main food groups when preparing snacks as well as main meals. A well-balanced mid-morning snack – say, three hours after breakfast – will provide a welcome, consistent energy boost and keep hunger at bay until lunchtime. By contrast, a bar of chocolate or a Danish pastry might give you a brief surge of energy, but it will soon wear off and you will be left feeling more hungry than ever.

It can be difficult to get sufficient fruit and vegetables from main meals alone, so it makes sense to use them as the basis for most of your snacks. Choose one fruit from the list on page 151 or one vegetable from the list on page 163 and use it as your starting point, then add a good source of

→

protein and maybe some complex carbs (although you can omit these). As a rough guide for portion size, the whole snack should fit neatly in the cupped palm of your hand.

Any combination will do, no matter how weird. So, if you fancy guava with cold roast beef, hummus with melon, or a rye cracker with tofu and leftover green beans, then go ahead! On the other hand, if you prefer more traditional snacks, the following list should provide more than enough inspiration to keep them interesting:

- Hummus with sliced peppers on an oatcake
- Apple or pear with a small piece of Cheddar or Gruyère cheese
- One plum with four walnuts
- Almond, cashew or peanut butter on a rye cracker or half a piece of toast
- Cottage cheese on corn cake
- A slice of leftover steak with five cherry tomatoes
- Mixed seeds and a small banana
- Half a teacup of cooked chickpeas with a teaspoon of Greek yoghurt, seasoned
- One tablespoon of plain yoghurt with blackberries
- Two slices of tempeh wrapped in lettuce leaves
- A slice of ham or smoked salmon with cos lettuce on an oatcake
- Feta cheese with celery crudités
- Small portion of salmon with sesame seeds and cucumber
- Boiled egg and mushrooms
- Sauerkraut on a cracker
- One tablespoon of cubed feta with diced radish
- A slice of leftover chicken or turkey with a raw chopped carrot

- A sardine mashed onto two oatcakes
- A kiwi fruit and four Brazil nuts
- Red pepper hummus with raw cauliflower crudités
- Mackerel pâté on a rye cracker
- Watermelon with mixed seeds
- A few cashew nuts and a peach
- Two teaspoons of avocado sprinkled with sunflower seeds
- Pickled herring on an oatcake
- Chicory leaves and a matchbox-sized block of Gouda

Assuming you will be eating between 2000 and 2500 calories a day, each snack should provide no more than 300 (and preferably closer to 200).

Afters

There is no easy way to say this, but I believe that desserts should be eaten only occasionally – maybe a maximum of once a week – or preferably not at all. This is because the typical dessert is an unhelpful combination of free sugar, starch, fat and unnecessary calories. For instance, a small serving of sticky toffee pudding contains around 200 calories, while a single scoop of chocolate ice cream has 135, not to mention 17g of fat, 11g of which are saturated.

In addition, their carb-heavy nature means that most desserts have the potential to upset the delicate balance between the major food groups that you should aim to maintain at every meal. Moreover, their refined sugars can increase inflammation, which can be detrimental to prostate health and cognitive function, and promote the growth of unfriendly bacteria in the gut, with all the problems that entails (see Chapter 10).

Sweets

Fruit is always an option if you feel you *have* to eat something sweet after a meal, and nutritionally it certainly has much more going for it than the likes of steamed puddings or tiramisu. A single apple, orange or pear contains beneficial fibre, antioxidants and other nutrients, and the same is true of a *small* portion (about enough to fill a teacup) of fruit salad.

However, fruit-based desserts are another matter entirely, as the fruit is just one of many ingredients, most of which are none too healthy. For example, apple crumble tends to be more crumble (a mixture of free sugars and starchy carbs) than apple.

Cheese

Opting for cheese after a meal, rather than something sweet, is one way of avoiding sugar, but it will have a similar impact on your calorie intake and could be even worse with regard to saturated fat.

Also, remember that you should limit your consumption of all dairy products to four servings each day, with the serving size for cheese no more than a matchbox-sized block.

Summary

You'll soon get the hang of choosing meals and snacks that are wholly consistent with the ManFood philosophy. However, we've covered a lot in this chapter, so here's a quick summary of the main points that you need to bear in mind:

- Always combine protein with complex carbs in the

form of grain/starch and vegetables (or just vegetables, if you prefer).

- The protein serving should be less than the size of your clenched fist, while the grains/starch should cover no more than the area of your fingers (held together) when your palm is turned upwards. The vegetable portion should cover your whole palm and thumb or more.

- An app can be useful in the early stages of the ManFood plan to provide information on calories and offer guidance on appropriate portion sizes (see the box on page 80). You should aim for no more than 2500 calories each day, with the two main meals each accounting for a maximum of 600–700.

- It's a good idea to eat lightly the day before and after a big event or celebration in order to compensate for the inevitable excess.

CHAPTER 15

Eating out

You may eat out only on special occasions, once a week, or almost every day (for instance, if your job demands it). Either way, it is still perfectly feasible to follow the ManFood plan even when you are not preparing the food yourself. Furthermore, you can afford the occasional lapse when eating out, as this will have little impact as long as you follow the guidelines for the majority of the time. You may want to think along the lines of 80:20 – adhere to the plan for 80 per cent of your meals, and you can allow yourself a bit more freedom for the remaining 20 per cent.

Remember, ManFood is not a strict, prescriptive, weight-loss programme. It's much more flexible than any diet plan. This means there's no wagon to fall off, so if you happen to have a big night out and overdo it, there's no need to slide into a spiral of self-recrimination and guilt. Just return to normal the next day by making yourself a healthy ManFood breakfast and continue from there.

Restaurant dining

Never forget that it is in the interests of every restaurant to provide delicious food that you will want to eat again. After all, their business depends on it. Consequently, they may use more salt and fat than you would ever dream of adding to a similar dish at home. They also want you to spend as much money as possible, so they'll try to tempt you with a range of starters and rich desserts, not to mention aperitifs and after-dinner drinks.

Nevertheless, eating out can still be a *healthy* experience as long as you make smart choices from the menu. Remember, you should eat a maximum of 6g of salt and 30g of saturated fat each day, so some care when ordering is always advisable. The following hints may prove helpful:

1. A single course from a restaurant is usually more than enough, but if you want more variety, why not choose two starters and eat one as your main course? This combination will probably contain fewer calories than any of the official main courses and should help you remain within the recommended limits for salt and fat, too.

2. There's no need to shun the bread basket, but if you do indulge, it's probably a good idea to steer clear of more starchy carbs during the main course. In other words, a large plate of spaghetti is not ideal if you've already had a couple of rolls.

3. Add butter or oil to the bread if you wish, but bear in mind that there is likely to be plenty in the dishes themselves, so keep it to a minimum. A knob of butter can contain 200 calories and would count as one of your four dairy portions for the day, while a thin scraping might be only 50g. Olive oil is preferable, not least because it contains polyphenols and vitamin E. However, rather than dipping the bread directly into the bowl, transfer a couple of teaspoons (about 80 calories) to your side plate and limit yourself to that.

4. Many restaurants offer starters and sides that they classify as 'healthy', such as 'superfood' salads. These are often good choices, especially if the restaurant allows the addition of a portion of grilled chicken breast or halloumi to convert the dish into a main course.

5. Sauces and dressings can be added quite liberally by busy kitchen staff, so order them on the side and exercise some discretion to limit your intake of salt, sugar and fat.

6. If you plan to drink, skip the aperitif and delay ordering the wine until your food has arrived. This is a simple way to reduce the speed with which your body absorbs the alcohol.

7. On the occasions when you do have a dessert, it's worth asking if any of your fellow diners would like to share. If you find a taker, you will cut your consumption of free sugars and saturated fat in half.

8. If you are eating later than your usual routine, it's wise to have a small snack an hour or two beforehand, as this will reduce the likelihood of overindulgence at the restaurant.

9. While protein is an important part of every meal in the ManFood plan, there's no need to include it in both your starter and your main course. Instead, choose an entirely vegetable option for the starter (or skip it altogether).

10. If you are unfamiliar with the venue, check the menu online beforehand. This will help you to make a smart, considered decision rather than a hurried, indiscriminate choice.

These tips should help you relax and enjoy a night out at the restaurant, safe in the knowledge that you are not veering too far from the ManFood ethos. But what should you order once you get there? Below, I suggest some healthy options for each of the most popular cuisines.

French

To start: asparagus or grilled vegetables, onion soup, fish soup or scallops. Main course: steak, grilled fish, rabbit, chicken casserole or duck, served with plenty of vegetables and possibly a few boiled new potatoes (rather than frites).

Italian

To start: bresaola or carpaccio (either fish or meat) with rocket, avocado, tomato and mozzarella, crab or seafood salad. Main course: veal, fish, calf's liver, beef or lamb, with vegetables. In addition, you could order a starter size of risotto to share. Alternatively, if you are part of a large group, share a pizza with the rest of the table, so you each get one slice.

Japanese

There's plenty of choice and most dishes – such as sashimi, grilled meats, poultry and cooked fish – can be eaten as either a starter or a main course, possibly with a small portion of brown rice as a side. This is also the perfect opportunity to boost your intake of probiotics with miso soup and pickled vegetables. Sushi is OK, but just be aware that it contains a lot of starchy white rice.

Chinese

Chinese food tends to be very carb-rich. For instance, dumplings and spring rolls are mostly dough and very little filling, and the portions of rice and noodles are often twice as large as they should be. Therefore, choose a soup to start, such as hot and sour, and follow with poultry, fish, tofu or meat, cooked simply, with a maximum of half a standard portion of rice or noodles.

Thai

Once again the focus is on carbs, although Thai rolls wrapped in rice paper are not fried, so they are a relatively healthy option, as are fishcakes and soup. A green or red curry with any protein (tofu, beef, fish, chicken, etc.) is a decent main course. Ask for vegetables on the side and, again, share a portion of rice or noodles. Note that coconut cream/milk is often used quite liberally in Thai cooking. This is mostly saturated fat, so it is advisable to avoid any dishes in which it is listed as one of the ingredients.

American

Beefburgers contain a lot of protein but also a large number of calories. For instance, a plain burger may provide over 500 calories, while the addition of cheese and bacon will push this up to 750 or more. Moreover, a small portion of fries will add a further 300. All of this is on top of the fact that burgers are not a particularly healthy option in the first place because, in itself, the bun provides too many starchy carbs. You can address this problem by throwing away the top half, but that would still leave a typical burger meal woefully short of vegetables.

Indian

To start: try to avoid or at least limit the fried dough choices and opt for vegetables, lentils or chickpeas instead. Poppadoms, which are made from lentil flour, are about 78 calories each, so be mindful if you order a stack for the table. Main course: tandoori meat or fish dishes are good options as they tend to be relatively plain, rather than swimming in sauce. Choose a rogan dish over one made with cream, as the former will have less saturated fat and contain tomato, ginger and garlic (all of which are good sources of antioxidants). Vegetarian choices, such as dishes consisting primarily of legumes or cheese, are usually on offer, too. However, watch the rice portions (share one between two or even three or your party) and bear in mind that even a plain naan can run to 500 calories, depending on the recipe.

DINNER PARTIES

Eating within certain parameters can be problematic when you are a guest in someone else's home, as you are unlikely to have much say in what appears on your plate. In addition, when family or friends make a meal, there can be a certain amount of social pressure to eat whatever is placed in front of you. A simple way round this is to request a small portion before the meal is served. In addition, if separate servings of vegetables form part of the meal, it's a good idea to load your plate with them in order to keep the ratio of complex carbs to protein as close as possible to ManFood guidelines.

Food on the go

Even with the best of intentions and careful preparation of healthy lunches and snacks, sometimes the only option is to grab something to eat on the go. This sort of food has a terrible reputation – think of motorway service-station pasties and burger vans – but it's not all bad. Indeed, many cafés, coffee shops and takeaways now offer surprisingly healthy options. In addition, there's a supermarket on nearly every high street, all of which stock basic ingredients from which you can cobble together something that is not only tasty but nutritious.

Breakfast

The following recommendations, which often come in small pots, are widely available in takeaway food outlets:

- Porridge with fruit, but forgo the honey and add a small sachet of nuts from the counter instead.
- Egg, avocado and spinach (or smoked salmon).
- Bircher muesli, but add some nuts and yoghurt.
- Egg, sausage and beans (not daily, due to the processed meat).
- Bacon and egg (not daily, as above), plus an apple if there are no vegetables in the pot.
- Fruit and granola, but this lacks protein so add some nuts or seeds.
- Salmon and egg muffin (although discard some of the muffin).

Avoid croissants, Danish pastries and compotes, as these are high in refined sugar and simple carbohydrates. In addition, the absence of fibre and protein means that they provide only a very short burst of energy and you will be hungry again within an hour or so. Of course, you could always add some cheese and/or ham to a croissant for their protein, although even this is not recommended on a regular basis as the meat is processed, the portion of cheese is likely to be excessively large, the number of calories and saturated fat content are too high and the fruit and vegetable content is still nil.

Lunch and more substantial meals

You will find a massive selection of wraps, salads and sandwiches on any high street, ranging from freshly prepared artisan rolls to the pre-packaged meal combos in large pharmacies. In light of this bewildering choice, here are a few pointers that should help you pick the best option:

- Wraps usually provide the most ManFood-friendly balance between the various food groups. Pick one with as many vegetables as possible and ensure that it contains some protein, too.
- Sandwiches are sometimes a little light on the filling, although a good old-fashioned sandwich shop will usually cram in some more if you ask politely. Any protein will do, but, as ever, don't neglect the vegetables. Opt for wholemeal, rye or granary bread.
- Bagels are fine, even better if you only eat half (they contain about 4g of fibre), but make sure they include some good protein and sliced vegetables.
- Pre-made sandwiches may not have adequate amounts of fibre or protein, but they are OK every once in a while if you have no other option. It is a good idea to add a small pot of edamame beans for a boost of complex carbs.

Salads provide many of the nutrients you need, especially if they contain crunchy vegetables as well as salad leaves. However, they may be a little light on the protein, so you could sprinkle a few seeds on top and have an oatcake on the side (or crumble it on top) for some extra fibre.

Vegetarian and vegan takeaway dishes mostly include protein in the form of beans, lentils or falafel – all of which are good choices. Soups are recommended, too, as they will almost invariably contain plenty of vegetables and protein.

Remember, you should aim for no more than 800 calories at lunch, which few on-the-go meals will exceed. However, if you add crisps, a fizzy drink and 'dessert' (such as a chocolate bar), you will go sailing beyond that figure. Standard crisps are never a good idea because they contain so much fat, and even the baked alternatives tend to be packed with excessive amounts of salt. A small pot of beans, coleslaw or vegetables is far preferable.

Sushi is widely available these days and provides healthy doses of omega 3 fats, selenium, vitamin B12 and potassium. There is also some fibre in the rice and seaweed as well as iodine in the latter. Salad leaves, edamame beans, avocado and spinach are also often found in sushi boxes, all of which will provide a welcome boost to your vegetable intake. If not, you can always add your own pot of edamame beans on the side.

Noodle and rice pots are tasty and usually offer some protein (such as chicken, salmon or tofu) along with plenty of vegetables. If there is a choice, opt for brown rice or wholewheat noodles, rather than white, for a little extra fibre.

Pies tend to contain far too much pastry, not enough filling and the salty, rich sauces are bad news, too. Therefore, as a general rule, they are not recommended. However, as with other poor choices, it's OK every once in a while.

Finally, remember that it is inadvisable to eat processed meat – such as bacon, sausages, ham and salami – every day, regardless of whether it is delivered in a sandwich, pie or wrap. Also, you should not exceed the maximum portion size of 50g when you do eat it.

From the supermarket

Instant oats provide a fibre-rich breakfast, but make sure you choose a plain variety as those with added ingredients invariably have added sugar, too. It's a simple enough task to add your own fruit and nuts (and none of the white stuff). Alternatively, you could grab a small pot of Greek yoghurt, a punnet of blueberries and a sachet of nuts, and combine them at work. (There'll be plenty of berries and nuts left over, which you can use as snacks later in the day.)

In addition to sandwiches and snacks, supermarkets offer dozens of decent lunch choices that require minimal preparation. Look for cooked but not processed meats – such as chicken or turkey – which are fine, although they do often contain a bit of added sugar. Cooked chicken fillets, some chopped vegetables and a pouch of cooked rice or quinoa may be kept in the office fridge overnight, so it can provide lunch over two consecutive days.

Canned fish and beans are other options, and both can be added to salads with vegetables and some grains. You'll also find dips – such as hummus, tzatziki and taramasalata – all of which contain some protein (hummus has the most). Eat with a pitta bread or crackers, or make some carrot or celery crudités.

A baked potato with beans is also acceptable, as long as you eat the skin for the extra fibre and don't pile too much cheese on top.

CHAPTER 16

Supplements

There's an unfortunate irony about supplements: the people who would benefit most from taking them – that is, those who do not eat a well-balanced diet for one reason or another – are the least likely to do so. Meanwhile, those who *do* eat healthy diets often spend a fortune on a whole host of unnecessary pills, tonics and tablets.

Supplement marketing tends to highlight the role of a specific nutrient, then presents the company's capsule or pill as the best means to get the recommended daily amount of that nutrient. Taken together, this twofold message can be compelling, because the company first focuses on the scientifically proven benefits of the nutrient – in terms of boosting your immune system, improving your heart health, protecting your bones or whatever – then implies that you are unlikely to get sufficient quantities of it from diet alone. However, it glosses over the fact that separating individual nutrients from food is, in a way, unnatural. Furthermore, swallowing the nutrients in isolation means that you lose the highly beneficial interplay between various vitamins and minerals, or fibre and fat, that you get when eating them together, in food form.

All that aside, though, do you really need to take supplements? Well, if you follow the ManFood plan and eat food that is rich in essential nutrients, the answer is probably 'No ... with one or two exceptions.' In addition, bear in mind that supplements may interfere with prescribed medication, so it's always advisable to check with your doctor or a professional nutritionist before investing in more (possibly unregulated) pills. (Incidentally, many GPs are sceptical about supplementation and may even suggest that it's simply a way to make 'expensive wee'. It's up to you whether you believe them or the supplement companies' claims and promises.)

Before starting any course of supplementation, you should be aware of the following:

1. As supplements come in pill or capsule form, you may feel like you are taking medication. However, their effects (if any) are rather more nebulous. For instance, if you have backache and take a couple of ibuprofen tablets, you will know that the medication has worked the moment the pain starts to subside. By contrast, if you take 100mg of vitamin C, this may do you some general good, but you will not be able to pinpoint a specific benefit.

2. Many supplements need to be taken consistently over the long term (maybe the rest of your life) to derive any significant benefit, which can prove expensive.

3. Quality is highly variable and some formulations use chemicals that are not easily absorbed. For instance, some calcium supplements contain calcium gluconate, which is 9 per cent elemental calcium (the amount of usable mineral in the formulation), whereas others contain calcium citrate, which might be as high as 21 per cent. Such differences tend to be reflected in the price, which is obviously an important consideration, as you will be taking them over the long term. This should be factored in when you make your decision about which brand to choose.

4. Supplements are active substances, so you *must* adhere to the recommended dosage on the package and/or advice from your GP or a professional nutritionist (*not* the sales assistant in the shop), if appropriate.

5. A few supplements may be taken tactically to address short-term issues. For instance, some may help if you have a cold or are constipated.

It could be argued that *every* nutrient could be taken in supplement form, because each plays so many important roles with regard to general health. Furthermore, given the potential advantages of boosting your intake of these beneficial compounds, and the absence of any significant drawbacks (aside from the long-term impact on your wallet), you may feel remiss if you do not take all of them, or possibly even reckless, especially if you go on to develop a condition that one or other may have prevented.

But where does it end? There are literally hundreds of different supplements on the market, so you would have to have a lot of time and money to take all of them each day for the rest of your life. More to the point, as mentioned earlier, a healthy, well-balanced diet makes large-scale supplementation unnecessary.

That said, especially once we reach middle age, there is certainly a case to be made for some limited supplementation. Below, I discuss many of the supplements you might already be taking (or are considering after reading this book) and whether it's really worth it. However, please note that all of the following recommendations are based on the assumption that you will be following the ManFood plan and therefore eating plenty of foods that are rich in the most important nutrients.

Supplements for the ManFood plan

Most men in their late forties and upwards would probably benefit from taking a small core group of supplements, plus one or two others, depending on individual circumstances.

You may notice that I don't recommend a standard multivitamin/mineral supplement. This is because they are unnecessary as long as you follow the dietary guidelines that are contained within this book. Nevertheless, perhaps you have been taking one for years and feel that you benefit from it. If so, that's fine – feel free to keep taking it. However, please check the label carefully to ensure that you do not go over the recommended daily amount for any nutrient by adding further supplements in response to the advice below.

In addition, if you are taking medication, it bears repeating that you should always consult with your GP before embarking on any course of supplementation, regardless of how benign it may seem.

In total, I believe it is worth considering nine supplements. These are listed in the table below, along with recommended daily dosage plus a rough indication of how beneficial each supplement may be. However, remember that we are all individuals, and all of our needs are different. So, for instance, if you work outside all year, you might have less need of a daily vitamin D tablet, especially in the summer. The subsequent detailed sections on each potential nutrient/supplement should help you make an informed decision that more closely reflects your particular circumstances and health requirements.

Supplement	Advisable	Probably beneficial	Possibly beneficial	Recommended daily dosage[†]
Vitamin D	✓			15–20mcg[‡]
Omega 3	✓			500mg
Vitamin B12	✓			100mcg
Magnesium		✓		200mg
Calcium		✓		<200mg
Selenium			✓	<200mcg
CoQ10			✓	100–200mg
Probiotics			✓	1 capsule
Digestive enzymes			✓	1 capsule

Notes: [†] This is the amount to be taken in supplement form. It is not the *total* recommended intake, which also encompasses food sources. For instance, the recommended daily intake of calcium for a man aged over 55 is 1200mg, but you will get most (if not all) of this from your food, assuming you eat dairy products, so you should usually limit your supplementation to a maximum of 200mg (see below for further details).
[‡] Micrograms are sometimes abbreviated as μg, rather than mcg, on supplement packaging.

Vitamin D

Health authorities in the UK and around the world recommend vitamin D supplementation. The recommended dosage for UK is 10mcg for adults and children alike, especially in autumn and winter, when sunlight is scarce.

As with all essential nutrients, vitamin D has a multitude of roles, including the maintenance of good prostate health and bone density, testosterone production and sleep promotion. It is not found in many foods, although oily fish and soya products (such as tofu and edamame beans) as well as shiitake and other mushrooms are reasonably good sources. There is also a small amount in egg yolks.

The amount of vitamin D in a pill or capsule is usually given in international units (iu). In the UK, the recommended daily dosage is 400iu – equivalent to 10mcg – assuming a diet that contains some vitamin D and some sun exposure. However, it may be advisable to take more in later years, when absorption from dietary sources may be impaired, and/or if you get less than fifteen minutes' direct sunlight most days. In addition, our ability to manufacture vitamin D from sunlight declines with age: by the age of 65 it may be down to a quarter of what it was in our twenties. Furthermore, men with dark skin have less capacity to produce vitamin D than those with paler skin. Also, vitamin D is fat soluble and can be stored away in fat cells, so overweight men are particularly vulnerable to deficiency. The solution is to lose weight and take a supplement.

Bearing all of this in mind, I suggest a daily dosage of 600–800iu (15–20mcg). The lower amount will be adequate if you get plenty of direct sun exposure every day, are pale-skinned, not overweight and eat vitamin D-rich foods on a regular basis. If any of these do not apply to you, increase the dosage to 800iu.

In particular, you should look for D3 – otherwise known as cholecalciferol – as it is especially effective. However, it is derived from sheep's wool so may be unsuitable if you follow a strict vegan lifestyle. In that case, you can use D2 – or ergocalciferol – instead.

Omega 3

There are three types of omega 3 fat – alpha linolenic acid (ALA), eicosapentaenoic acid (EPA) and docosahexaenoic acid (DHA).

ALA is found in soya beans, walnuts, flaxseeds (or linseeds), pumpkin seeds, chia seeds and hemp seeds, as well as their respective oils. Purslane is another good source, and it is also found in somewhat smaller quantities in many leafy green vegetables. However, while ALA is considered an essential fat, most of the potential benefits of omega 3 fats are derived from EPA and DHA. Oily fish, such as mackerel, pilchards, kippers, sardines, salmon, whitebait, herring and swordfish, is the richest source of both, and they are also found in crab meat.

As we have seen throughout this book, these essential fats play many important roles in human health, such as helping to combat cognitive decline (see Chapter 3), alleviating insulin resistance (Chapter 5) and reducing inflammation (Chapter 7).

If you eat oily fish three or four times a week, as recommended in the ManFood plan, each serving probably provides about 450mg of both EPA and DHA, but there is still a case for taking a daily 500mg omega 3 capsule, especially on those days when you don't eat fish. Choose an 'omega 3' – rather than simply a 'fish oil' – supplement. Alternatively, especially if you follow a vegetarian or vegan lifestyle, opt for a supplement that is derived from algae, as these offer EPA and DHA, rather than the less beneficial ALA.

However, it should be noted that all fat supplements should be avoided if you are taking medication that may increase bleeding, such as blood thinners or drugs to prevent blood clots, as well as non-steroidal anti-inflammatories (NSAIDS), such as ibuprofen, aspirin and naproxen, all of which are common painkillers. If you take any of these medications regularly, you must consult your GP before supplementing omega 3.

Vitamin B12

Vitamin B12 is plays a crucial role in many of the body's most important functions, including energy production, homocysteine production, maintaining the coating that surrounds and protects the nerves and melatonin production. It is bound to proteins in food but released from these in the stomach due to the activity of hydrochloric acid and the enzyme gastric protease. Thereafter, it combines with intrinsic factor, a substance produced by certain cells in the lining of the stomach, and the new compound is then absorbed.

However, levels of hydrochloric acid may fall as we age, potentially hindering this process and reducing our ability to obtain B12 from food. Absorption is also affected by digestive disorders and pernicious anaemia. However, B12 is stored in the liver, so it may be some time before this problem becomes apparent.

B12 in supplement form is not bound to protein, so absorption is not so reliant on digestive capability. Nevertheless, B12 assimilation can be limited if there is more B12 than the intrinsic factor can accommodate.

B12 is found naturally in liver, red meat, poultry, game, oily fish, eggs and dairy products (especially fermented ones, such as yoghurt and kefir). As these foods feature prominently in the ManFood plan, you may not need to take a supplement at the moment. However, your need may increase as you age, given that stomach acid tends to decline significantly from the age of 55 onwards.

Some cereals, soya and nut milks and juices are fortified with B12, in part because there are no natural plant-based sources, but supplementation may still be beneficial if you follow a vegetarian or vegan lifestyle.

Supplements are widely available in spray, capsule and patch form. These tend to contain far higher doses than the very modest recommended daily amount of 2.5mcg because they are designed to overcome what may be extreme problems with B12 absorption. Dosages range from 100 to 1000mcg, although the lower figure is usually more than adequate.

B12 is also often included in so-called 'B complex' supplements, which combine several B vitamins in a single capsule or tablet. Once again, the average daily dose is 100mcg. (Note that most B complex supplements contain B2, or riboflavin, which turns urine bright yellow. This is quite normal and no cause for alarm.)

Oral sprays tend to provide much higher doses – usually in the region of 1200mcg. Moreover, the liquid is sprayed under the tongue, which means it is absorbed quickly. Some popular brands suggest four sprays a day, but it is highly unlikely that you would need any more than two.

Patches are high strength, too – usually around 1000mcg. The instructions generally recommend applying and leaving on the skin for twenty-four hours, once a week (although some brands suggest twice a week). I feel that one patch per week would provide ample B12 for most people.

Magnesium

Magnesium plays an important role in improving sleep patterns, reducing stress, boosting testosterone production and maintaining bone density, especially from middle age onwards. It is found naturally in oat bran, brown rice, quinoa, pumpkin and sunflower seeds, wholegrains, nuts, lentils and dark green leafy vegetables, yet many older UK men are still magnesium deficient.

The recommended total daily intake is 375mg. A small (30g) serving of oats will provide around 55mg, 30g of spinach 34mg and 28g of cooked brown rice only 12mg. Given these modest amounts in even the best sources, taking a magnesium supplement may be beneficial. A dose of 200mg an hour before bedtime may improve your sleep if you suffer from insomnia. If this is not an issue, then it may be better to take the supplement every other day, with your evening meal.

Note that some widely prescribed medications for peptic ulcers, acid reflux, water retention and even some antibiotics react with magnesium, so you should consult your GP if you are taking any of these. If you are prescribed a course of antibiotics, it is advisable to suspend magnesium supplementation for the whole course and the following week.

Calcium

Although calcium plays a pivotal role in maintaining bone density, excess calcium is potentially a risk factor for prostate cancer. Therefore, it's important to keep your total intake at just the right level. As we have seen, the recommended daily amount is 800mg a day for younger men, but this rises to 1000–1200mg for those over the age of 55. If you eat dairy products, most of this will be provided by your diet.

The ManFood plan recommends a maximum of four modest servings of dairy each day (for instance, a matchbox-sized block of cheese, a small yoghurt and milk in tea and coffee), but if you also eat broccoli, kale, beans, almonds, sesame seeds and/or soft fish (sardines and whitebait), you should be getting sufficient calcium from food sources alone.

Therefore, if you do decide to take a supplement, a daily dose of less than 200mg will probably suffice. On the other hand, if you do not eat dairy products, have a digestive condition (such as coeliac disease), favour a high-protein diet or eat in excess of 6g of salt each day, you may need more. The same may be true if you have been diagnosed with osteoporosis, but this is a matter that you should discuss with your doctor.

Selenium

Men require some 25 per cent more of this mineral than women, because some of the body's reserves are lost during each ejaculation. Therefore, if you are sexually active, it is advisable to eat a selenium-rich diet or, if necessary, take a supplement. This is because selenium supports liver function and is one of the key components of glutathione perixodase -- a potent antioxidant that is especially important in protecting the cardiovascular system, maintaining cognitive function and ensuring good prostate health. It is found naturally in offal, herring, Brazil nuts and mushrooms, although levels vary considerably depending on the environment in which the produce was grown or the animals grazed.

On average, a single Brazil nut contains some 79.5mcg. Therefore, if you are partial to these nuts, you should be extremely careful, as the *maximum* daily allowance of selenium is just 400mcg. (By contrast, the *recommended* daily allowance is a mere 55mcg.) Of course, this limit must be respected if you choose to take a selenium supplement, so I would recommend a maximum dose of 200mcg, preferably 100mcg, given that you will probably get some from your diet, too. Also remember to check general supplements – such as multivitamins and antioxidant complexes – as some of them contain selenium. An excess of selenium in the body is known as selenosis; symptoms include nausea, diarrhoea, mood swings and breathing problems.

CoQ10

If you have recently been prescribed a statin to manage your cholesterol, then you may be suffering from myopathy (muscle cramps, spasms and weakness). This may be linked to the fact that statins inhibit the body's ability to produce co-enzyme Q10. Myopathy usually passes after a few uncomfortable weeks, but in some cases it can persist.

Co-enzyme Q10 – commonly known as CoQ10 – is a nutrient that not only plays a role in the body's energy-making process but also has antioxidant properties. Moreover, levels fall naturally as we age, so there is certainly an argument for taking a supplement after middle age, especially if you are on statins. However, while a number of studies have suggested that CoQ10 supplementation is a worthwhile investment, others have found no tangible benefits.

Your doctor or cardiologist will probably try a different type of statin if you experience long-term myopathy. If this doesn't alleviate the symptoms, however, then it is certainly worth discussing the merits of supplementing 100–200mg of CoQ10 per day.

Probiotics

As we saw in Chapter 10, gut bacteria – be they 'good' or 'bad', and the balance between the two – have a profound influence on many aspects of human health, including irritable bowel syndrome, food intolerance and sensitivity, bone density, weight gain and loss, appetite, energy, atherosclerosis, inflammation, arthritis and autoimmune conditions. They may even play a role in depression.

In the same chapter, we also saw that fermented foods – such as kefir, miso, kombucha and yoghurt – increase the numbers of good bacteria in the gut. However, many of these foods will be unfamiliar and indeed an acquired taste that you have no wish to acquire. If that's the case, it may be worth considering a probiotic supplement. (Although, as ever, food sources are preferable.)

Look for brands that contain various strains of *Lactobacillus* and *Bifidobacterium* (most do). The usual recommended dosage is a single capsule once a day, but if your diet includes probiotic foods and/or prebiotics (such as chicory, onions and Jerusalem artichokes), every second or third day will suffice.

Digestive enzymes

As previously mentioned, production of hydrochloric acid and therefore digestive capacity decline with age, with one estimate suggesting a 30 per cent reduction by the age of 60. Obviously, this impairs the body's ability to absorb many of the nutrients that are found in food, so taking a supplement that increases the level of stomach acid may seem more logical – and cost-effective – than supplementing all of the nutrients themselves.

Symptoms of poor digestion that may be linked to lower levels of stomach acid include cracked or weak nails, flatulence, belching and undigested food in the stool. If you suffer from any of these complaints, it might be worth taking a digestive enzyme supplement that contains hydrochloric acid (check the label, as some do not). These supplements must always be taken with food, as the acid they contain can cause discomfort and even pain if they are taken on an empty stomach.

FOOD-BASED SUPPLEMENTS

Although you can get almost all of the nutrients you need from the recommended foods in the ManFood plan, you may feel the need for an occasional boost. Fortunately, there is something of a halfway house between no supplements at all and a long-term supplementation regime in the form of food-based products that contain concentrated amounts of certain nutrients.

A few years ago, these might have been dubbed 'super-foods', but in truth there is no such thing. They are simply a different form of supplementation that you can add to your regular meals, snacks and drinks as and when you please. For example, you could add a teaspoon of matcha powder and/or turmeric to smoothies, fruit juice or kefir for a large, instant hit of nutrients such as curcumin, catechins and antioxidants. Alternatively, there are many fruit- and vegetable-based manufactured powders on the market.

I should stress that you won't 'need' any of these products if you follow the ManFood plan (and take one or two conventional supplements, if necessary). They are very much optional extras. That said, I do believe they have some merit and even use some of them myself, on occasion.

Bear in mind that a number of important nutrients, including vitamins D, A, K and E and some carotenoids, are fat-soluble, so absorption rates will be compromised if the powder itself contains no fat and you add it to a fat-free foodstuff.

Finally, protein powders and shakes are almost certain to be surplus to requirements if you follow the basic principles of the ManFood plan. They may provide a tiny amount of benefit after weight-bearing exercise, but really you should be getting more than enough protein from your diet alone.

My personal supplement routine

I took a vast array of nutrients when I started studying nutrition in the mid-1990s, even though I ate quite well. However, as I learned more, it eventually dawned on me that the vast majority of them were superfluous, so I cut the number dramatically.

You won't be surprised to learn that I still eat a healthy, well-balanced diet, but I am twenty years older. All of our needs change as we age, and I am no exception. I also have coeliac disease, which may impair the absorption of certain nutrients, even though, by necessity, my diet is gluten free.

With that information in mind, my supplement routine is as follows:

- Daily: vitamin D, omega 3, B complex.
- Every few days: probiotic capsule.
- When required: magnesium before bed (to aid sleep).
- If I feel I have a cold coming on: 15mg of zinc citrate twice a day for no more than a few days (it is not advisable to take this amount of zinc for extended periods of time); 250mg of olive-leaf extract, again for a few days. (The evidence for the efficacy of both of these supplements is far from conclusive, which is why I have not mentioned them earlier in this chapter. However, this combination seems to work for me.)

CHAPTER 17

Final thoughts

I am in my mid-fifties and the years appear to be sliding by more quickly than I care for. It seems like only last week that I was 50, yet 60 is now on the horizon. Getting older has some welcome rewards, of course, but there are challenges too, not least with the health issues that typically face men as we age.

I want to do everything I can to sail through the years to come in the best of health and, to my mind, there is no better place to start than with nutrition. The reason for this is not simply because all of us eat, and making choices that can serve us well now, and in the future, makes sense, but also because nutrition plays a vital role in how we feel and function. In that sense, what you have read in the preceding pages has a personal element to it, because when I was researching and writing *ManFood* I was reminded once again of the central role that nutrition has in creating optimal health. Despite being a nutritional therapist who has a largely good diet, I found there were areas that I could improve on without too much effort.

Unfortunately, nutrition has become overly complicated, as foods go in and out of fashion, often without robust evidence to support the dramatic headlines and news reports. *ManFood* cuts through all that and deals with the important health issues that we all face, without waffle or pseudoscience, explaining exactly how nutrition can help reduce our chances of being affected by the conditions that typically arise as we grow older. Making simple changes to your diet, swapping this food for that, or eating more of something you already eat, can go a long way to offset such conditions. As you have discovered, the nutrients I have highlighted and the foods they are found in aren't exotic and strange, rather they are found in many of the familiar foods you are probably already eating, along with a few that you maybe should be.

Most importantly, I believe that the advice, tips and guidance in *ManFood* are practical and easy to follow and that the foods are enjoyable. Given how simple it can be, I encourage you to adopt as many of the habits that you can. You might want to think about nutrition like a pension plan – you are doing your bit now to provide the best for yourself in the coming years.

If you have questions then I will do my best to reply in a timely fashion, although time won't allow great detail, you can find me at ianmarber.com and also on Twitter, @IanMarber. If you would like a personal consultation, or details of references, please get in touch via my website.

Sample menu plan

The week-long plan overleaf has been carefully created to include all the dietary elements that I've been encouraging you to eat in the preceding pages. If you were to deconstruct the foods for each day you'd find that the meaningful nutrients are represented daily, but, more importantly, the food suggestions are all easy, tasty and practical. That is the essence of the ManFood plan – foods that deliver on nutrients but are delicious and convenient. Naturally, some foods won't suit everyone, so you can make changes, as long as you swap the food with something similar.

	Monday	**Tuesday**	**Wednesday**
Breakfast	Porridge made with milk, chopped plum, walnuts	Poached egg, granary toast with avocado	Wholegrain cereal (Oatbix or Weetabix) with milk, toasted seeds and banana
Snack	Hummus with sliced red pepper	Cashew nuts and a peach	Almond butter on two oatcakes
Lunch	Chicken breast, salad leaves, broccoli, cucumber, tomato, avocado with olive oil, garlic, lemon juice dressing	Hummus salad sandwich with sliced tomato and lettuce on granary or rye bread	Salmon and tuna sushi, seaweed, edamame beans
Snack	Greek yoghurt with blackberries	Parmesan cheese and a pear	Kiwi fruit and Brazil nuts
Dinner	Blackened salmon, sweet potato, asparagus, baked kale	Miso soup followed by baked chicken leg, cherry tomatoes and garlic, with black beans stirred in for the last five minutes	Onion soup followed by lentil curry made with tomato, cauliflower, garlic and turmeric with brown rice

Thursday	Friday	Saturday	Sunday
Greek yoghurt, blueberries, blackberries, walnuts	Smoked salmon, cream cheese on wholewheat toast or half a toasted wholewheat bagel	Omelette, peppers, mushrooms and spring onion	Sausage, baked beans, poached egg and granary toast
Apple and Gouda cheese	Guacamole with carrot	Salmon pâté with an oatcake	Taramasalata on an oatcake
Rib-eye steak, baked potato, grilled tomato, spinach, leeks	Vegetable soup, such as tomato, broccoli, onion, etc., cannellini beans and grated Parmesan with an oatcake crumbled on top	Lamb chops, ratatouille, quinoa, green beans	Roast lamb, red cabbage, two roast potatoes, spinach
Oatcakes and tuna pâté	Tahini on mini pitta bread	Feta cheese and celery	Apricot and mixed seeds with a spoonful of plain yoghurt
Grilled sardines, sauerkraut, new potato	Calf's liver, broad beans, red cabbage and mashed sweet potato	Tricolore salad with avocado, tomato and mozzarella followed by seafood pasta and salad with cauliflower, broccoli, cucumber and a garlic/olive oil/ balsamic vinegar dressing	Squash soup with black beans

Store cupboard essentials

The right tools are essential if you want to do a job properly. With respect to the ManFood plan, this means ensuring that you have a well-stocked store cupboard that contains most – if not all – of the following foodstuffs.

Beans

Canned in plain water, without any added sugar or salt.

- Cannellini beans
- Black beans
- Chickpeas
- Butter beans
- Green lentils
- Black lentils
- Kidney beans

Nut butters

Roasted with no sugar (and preferably no salt or oil) added.

- Almond
- Cashew
- Peanut
- Brazil nut
- Hazelnut

Fish and seafood

Tinned in plain water, oil or (unsweetened) tomato sauce.

- Tuna
- Salmon
- Pilchards
- Sardines
- Mackerel

- Anchovies
- Cockles
- Mussels
- Oysters
- Crab meat

Nuts and seeds

Plain, roasted or raw, not salted or caramelised.

- Brazil nuts
- Hazelnuts
- Cashews
- Pistachios

- Sesame seeds
- Pumpkin seeds
- Chia seeds
- Almonds

Herbs and spices

Fresh or dried in bottles.

- Black peppercorns
- Long pepper
- Red peppercorns
- Oregano
- Rosemary
- Turmeric
- Cumin seeds

- Peri-peri powder
- Onion salt
- Garlic flakes
- Basil
- Parsley
- Mint
- Lemongrass

- Chopped ginger
- Italian seasoning
- Chives
- Tomato paste
  and passata
- Hot chilli powder
  and flakes
- Paprika
  (regular and hot)

- Dried roe (usually
  mullet, to grate over
  eggs and vegetables)
- Saffron
- Stock cubes,
  powder or paste
- Dried seaweed
  strips or flakes

Grains

- White rice
- Brown rice
- Wild rice
- Red rice

- Wholewheat pasta
- Rice noodles
- Quinoa

Sauces

- Mustard
- Hot sauce

- Horseradish sauce
- Lemon juice

Oils

- Extra-virgin olive oil
- Toasted
  sesame-seed oil
- Truffle oil

- Walnut oil
- Flavoured olive oil
  (such as lemon, garlic
  or chilli)

Index

Acknowledgements

With grateful thanks to: Amanda Preston at LBA for her persistence; Kieran Smith for his patience; everyone at Little, Brown for their guidance, especially Jillian Stewart and Emily Arbis; and to my friends and colleagues in the nutrition and dietetic community for their support and encouragement.